America's #1 Choice for Healthy Living

ENERGY BOOSTERS

By the Editors of *Prevention* Health Books

RODALE

ST. MARTIN'S
PAPERBACKS

Notice
This book is intended as a reference volume only, not as a medical manual. The information given here is designed to help you make informed decisions about your health. It is not intended as a substitute for any treatment that may have been prescribed by your doctor. If you suspect that you have a medical problem, we urge you to seek competent medical help.

The information in this book is excerpted from *Energy for Everything: Rejuvenation for the Mind, Body, and Soul* (Rodale, 2001).

Prevention's Best is a trademark and *Prevention* Health Books is a registered trademark of Rodale Inc.

ENERGY BOOSTERS

© 2001 by Rodale Inc.

Cover Designer: Anne Twomey
Book Designer: Keith Biery

ISBN 0–312–97879–0   paperback

Printed in the United States of America

Rodale/St. Martin's Paperbacks edition published September 2001

St. Martin's Paperbacks are published by St. Martin's Press, 175 Fifth Avenue, New York, NY 10010.

10 9 8 7 6 5 4 3 2

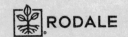

RODALE

WE **INSPIRE** AND **ENABLE** PEOPLE TO IMPROVE
THEIR LIVES AND THE WORLD AROUND THEM

Lila Amdurska Wallis, M.D., M.A.C.P.
Clinical professor of medicine at Weill Medical College of Cornell University in New York City, past president of the American Medical Women's Association (AMWA), founding president of the National Council on Women's Health, director of continuing medical education programs for physicians, and Master and Laureate of the American College of Physicians

Carla Wolper, M.S., R.D.
Nutritionist and clinical coordinator at the Obesity Research Center at St. Luke's–Roosevelt Hospital Center and nutritionist at the Center for Women's Health at Columbia Presbyterian Eastside, both in New York City

Contents

Introduction

Do you find yourself coveting sleep the way some women crave chocolate? Or fantasizing about checking into a hotel room alone and sleeping for a solid week? If so, you're not alone. "More energy" ranks right up there with "more time" and "more money" on a lot of women's wish lists.

Fatigue is one of the top 10 complaints—if not *the* top complaint—that send women to their doctors.

No wonder. Consider a typical day one woman described to us: Up at 6, walk the dog, get the kids up and dressed, make various and sundry breakfasts and lunches, walk the dog (again), drive to work, cram 12 hours of work into 8 (if she's lucky), reverse the commute, get the kids, chauffeur to soccer practice, do the dinner rush, clean the kitchen, fold the laundry, pay the bills, and—oh, yeah—try to remember to talk to that man in the corner who's her husband. Just writing it all down is exhausting.

If this description sounds like a carbon copy of your life, this book can help. It will show you how to change your work habits, employ less labor-intensive ways to clean your house, boost your energy through the magic of exercise, and develop more get-up-and-go than a triple espresso.

But this is more than a self-help book. It's told through the experiences of a modern "everywoman" named Carolyn, who, like most of us, is exhausted. As you read this book, you'll follow Carolyn throughout her hectic life—to work, her kids' soccer games, the supermarket, even the gym. In chapter after chapter, you'll watch as she integrates into her life the ideas and tips crammed throughout the book, eventually becoming a more energetic, relaxed, *alive* person.

This book will provide you with ideas for energy-enhancing foods as well as specific exercises you can do at your desk, or at a stoplight, to beat the afternoon doldrums. It will show you how to get your husband and kids to help with the housework, how to corral those mounds of energy-sapping clutter into order, and how to do something you thought only children did: play.

It will help you reinvigorate yourself, in the process improving your health, reducing your stress, and smoothing out the wrinkles of your life.

Ready to find this new, lively you? Just turn the page.

PART ONE

Where Did All the Energy Go?

Meet Carolyn: She's Everywoman and She's Exhausted

It's 6:15 P.M. Carolyn, a 49-year-old mother of two, walks in the door, throws her keys on the hallway table, and ponders one of Modern Woman's most perplexing dilemmas: cook or get takeout?

It's a no-brainer. Her husband, Ben, an engineer who travels frequently, is in Ohio for the next few days. Anyway, her kids—Jocelyn, 13, in 7th grade, and Michael, 16, in 10th grade—would rather have pizza.

She wearily reaches for the phone. As usual, she's exhausted.

Give Carolyn a choice between chocolate, sex, and a long, delicious nap, and she will invariably choose the snooze. Her go-go schedule at work, equally demanding kids, and ailing mother keep her on the run from 6 A.M., when she rises, to 11:30 or 12 at night, when she puts away the vacuum cleaner.

The worst part: With her husband away much of the time, she's often forced to tackle the unremitting demands of modern life solo.

If you're shaking your head at Carolyn's plight, save some sympathy for yourself. Fatigue among women is, in fact, an epidemic. Women—especially those in the child-bearing years—complain of fatigue more often than men. Let's call it female fatigue syndrome, or FFS.

This tiredness isn't just physical, however. Research suggests that women's fatigue is a slippery condition with many intertwining causes, both biological (such as menstruation and menopause) and psychological (such as stress and depression). The sweeping social changes that have occurred in recent decades in the workplace, our families, and our lifestyles also contribute to FFS.

Let's take a closer look at Carolyn's life to find out why she is so darn drained.

Round One: Carolyn Goes to Work

As an executive assistant to the president of a software company, Carolyn has a demanding full-time job, including long hours and high stress. She's wired—and not just emotionally. Armed with cell phone and pager, she practically beeps and chirps as she walks.

It's not unusual for her boss to call her at 10 P.M. Or for her to take work home. Which she dutifully completes, unless she falls asleep on the sofa at 8:30 in front of her favorite sitcom.

Bet you can relate.

Women have *always* worked, whether on the farm or in the home. But today an unprecedented number of us find ourselves locked in to the 40-hour-plus workweek.

And we're not only working but also working more. A 1998 national survey conducted by the Families and

Work Institute in New York City found that women worked an average of 44 hours a week—an increase of 5 hours a week since 1977. Another large study conducted by the same organization found that 68 percent of working parents with children under age 6 said their jobs required them to work very long and very hard—up from 55 percent in 1977.

The Dilemma of the Single Mom

Nearly 10 million women in the United States are raising children alone. If you're one, the worries and frustrations that come with the territory can drain you. The following tips from Andrea Engber, founder of the National Organization of Single Mothers and author of *The Complete Single Mother*, can help stoke your energy.

Make time for you. No matter what it takes. You'll wear out completely if you try to handle all the tasks of single parenting without taking a break now and then.

Make your own family rules. Abandon all hope of perfection. Do what works for you and your kids. When you're beat, ignore the clutter. If you're too tired to cook, serve peanut butter on whole-grain bread, or pancakes and fresh fruit.

Buy an egg timer. Set it for 20 minutes and tell your kids you're taking a timeout. Use the time to read, talk to a friend on the phone, surf the Net—whatever jump-starts your energy.

Nix the guilt. Repeat this mantra: I Can Do Only the Best I Can. Eventually, you'll come to believe it. For more information on the National Organization of Single Mothers, check out its Web site at www.singlemothers.org.

One study looked at moms in 1965, who primarily stayed home, and moms in 1998, who primarily worked outside the home, and found that both sets spent about the same amount of time with their children. How could that be? The moms in 1998 were taking time away from themselves. They slept 5 to 6 hours less per week and had 11 to 12 hours less free time for themselves per week.

Here's the irony: As our working hours have increased, so, too, has our sense that at work we sometimes feel more competent, more appreciated, and even more relaxed than we feel at home. Fact is, household and family obligations can make "home" work harder—and more frustrating— than paid work.

Eminent sociologist Arlie Russell Hochschild, D.Ph., Ph.D., of the University of California at Berkeley, spent three summers studying a company that offered "family-friendly policies," such as job sharing, part-time work, and telecommuting from home. What she found: Few men and women took advantage of them.

In the book based on her research, *The Time Bind: When Work Becomes Home and Home Becomes Work*, Dr. Hochschild notes that one out of five workers preferred paid office work to handling frustrating family and household obligations. She writes, "Nowadays, men and women both may leave unwashed dishes, crying tots, testy teenagers, and unresponsive mates behind to arrive at work early."

Round Two: Carolyn Goes on "Second Shift"

When Ben is at home—which isn't often—he's glad to be there. It's his sanctuary from the cares of the modern world.

But not Carolyn's.

As soon as she steps through the front door, her second shift begins—cooking dinner, refereeing the kids' squabbles, doing laundry.

The "second shift" refers to the long hours of family and household obligations we attend to before and after our "real" jobs. In *The Second Shift: Working Parents and the Revolution at Home*, Dr. Hochschild calculated that women with full-time jobs who also did housework and child care worked about 15 hours a week more than men—an extra month each year.

Sometimes the shift starts before we get home. Carolyn needs to ferry her kids to and from piano and ballet lessons as well as baseball and soccer games, necessitating an elaborate arrangement of car pools, shortened workdays, and favors begged of the neighbors.

Women didn't volunteer for the second shift. So why are we doing it?

In part because of the feminist movement in the 1970s, when we made great inroads into the labor market. In the early days of feminism, "we accepted the career template that had been designed for men," says Phyllis Moen, Ph.D., a sociologist at Cornell University in Ithaca, New York, and director of the Cornell Employment and Family Careers Institute. So while we gained equal opportunity, "we were still playing by men's rules," she says. "Which means that we also had the 'right' to work 60 or 70 hours a week. And yet, on the domestic front, nothing was taken off the plate."

In 1965, we spent 27 hours a week on housework; in 1995, 15.6 hours. But even being more relaxed about housekeeping can't make up for what we *really* need—a major rethinking of the traditional career path.

"Family-friendly work policies are merely window dressing around the old-style male career model," says Dr.

Moen. "We need to reinvent career paths that acknowledge that most workers—male or female—have family responsibilities."

Round Three: Carolyn Cares for Mom

Several times a week, Carolyn makes the 15-mile run out to her mother's house. Since her mother's health began to fail, Carolyn has been doing the older woman's laundry, buying her groceries, and visiting to keep her spirits up, often for as long as 2 hours.

Carolyn's care of her mother is mirrored by an estimated 22 million caregiving households in America, triple the number in 1988. The most recent report of family caregiving in this country—conducted by the National Alliance for Caregiving and the American Association of Retired Persons—paints a vivid picture of the typical caregiver (73 percent of caregivers are female).

The typical caregiver is a married woman in her mid-forties who works full-time. Moreover, 41 percent of all caregivers, male or female, have one or more children under 18 years old in the house.

Carolyn's lucky—she's not a "level 5" caregiver, defined as someone who provides constant care, or 40 or more hours of care per week. But even "part-time" caregivers like Carolyn, who are at level 3 (providing 9 hours of care per week), can experience some stress and fatigue, says Gail Hunt, executive director of the National Alliance for Caregiving in Bethesda, Maryland. And the burden doesn't decrease even when an ailing parent moves into a care facility, such as a nursing home, says Hunt.

"Many women drive over to feed their parents," Hunt says. "And when we do focus groups, we hear all the time

Pay Your Debt!

We're talking about sleep debt—or sleep deprivation—which is losing significant chunks of sack time for nights, weeks, or even months. As many as 80 percent of Americans experience it. The consequences go far beyond making us look like death warmed over.

In one study, men allotted 4 hours of sleep for 6 straight nights showed changes in thyroid function and metabolism. The researchers suggested that chronic sleep loss might also worsen certain age-related conditions, such as diabetes and high blood pressure.

To find out how much debt you've racked up, heed the signs—becoming drowsy or falling asleep while watching TV, driving, or reading a book. Another sign: irritability, says James Walsh, M.D., executive director of the Unity Sleep Medicine and Research Center at St. Luke's Hospital in Chesterfield, Missouri, and vice president of the National Sleep Foundation.

To repay your debt, try taking a simple nap, suggests Dr. Walsh. "It won't interfere with your sleep unless you nap for more than an hour or two during the day or close to your bedtime."

You'll know you've paid back your sleep debt when you can sit down in front of the TV or read a book and be bored rather than sleepy, Dr. Walsh says.

about women who get calls at 3 A.M. from the facility: 'We can't deal with her. She's all upset. You have to come over.'"

In the report, when caregivers were asked what kind of help or support they most wanted, the answer was, not surprisingly, "time for myself." That desire even beat out "help with housework" and extra money or financial support.

Round Four: Carolyn Takes a "Relaxing" Bath

It's 10:25 P.M. Carolyn has just finished unloading the dishwasher, folding the laundry, and paying bills. The kids are silent. The house is silent. Before her stretches a brief, shining gap of time before the grind begins again.

It's Carolyn Time.

She pads into the bathroom and fills the tub with warm water and lavender-scented bubble bath. (She's read that the scent of lavender helps reduce stress, and she needs all the help she can get.)

As she soaks, her mind relaxes . . . then suddenly recoils.

Will her mother eventually need to be moved to a nursing home? If so, how will they afford it?

Will she and Jocelyn bridge the ever-widening gap between them? As luck would have it, her daughter is entering puberty just as Carolyn is on the cusp of menopause, both intensely stressful transitions. While Carolyn knows that her daughter needs patience and support now, the constant bickering between them is wearing her down.

Will she and Ben ever have sex again? They've both been exhausted.

Will she make the deadline for the report due next Wednesday?

She drains the tub, feeling drained herself. But not sleepy. She knows it will be hours before she falls asleep.

Stress and its kin insomnia are major causes of fatigue. From 1985 to 1990, the proportion of people who reported "feeling highly stressed" more than doubled. And on an average workday, 1 million workers stay home because of stress-related complaints.

Carolyn *wishes* she could stay home—to sleep. Whether because of worrying into the wee hours or a dawn-till-dusk schedule, she sleeps only about 6 hours a night.

It's hard to believe that in 1910, the era of ragtime and mutton-sleeved blouses, the typical American slept an average of 9 hours a night. These days, we get an average of 7 hours. And in a recent poll conducted by the National Sleep Foundation, 45 percent of respondents admitted that they sleep less to accomplish more.

How Tired Are You?

Rate how likely you'd be to nod off in the following situations. Give yourself no points if you'd never doze off, 1 point for a slight chance, 2 for a moderate chance, and 3 for a high chance.

Sitting and reading

Watching television

Sitting as a passenger in a car for an hour without a break

Lying down to rest in the afternoon

Sitting and talking to someone

Sitting quietly after a lunch without alcohol

Sitting in a car, stopped for a few minutes in traffic

Scoring

0–5 points: slight or no sleep debt

6–10 points: moderate sleep debt

11–20 points: heavy sleep debt

21–25 points: extreme sleep debt

Accomplish more—but give ourselves less.

In 1977, working moms spent 96 minutes per workday on themselves. By the turn of the century, that precious hour and a half shrank to just 54 minutes, according to the Families and Work Institute study.

What we couldn't do with those 42 long, luscious lost minutes!

Round Five: Carolyn Loses It—And Finds an Answer

It's 11:18 P.M. Carolyn is in front of the TV, waiting for the news to end so she can doze off to the soothing banter of Jay Leno. But she knows that tomorrow is going to be a killer, especially on 5½ hours of sleep.

A tear rolls down her cheek. Then another.

"I just can't face it. I just can't," she thinks.

She remembers how her life used to be—when she wasn't so tired, when she wasn't working 45 hours a week, when she and Ben and the kids would just pile into the minivan on a Saturday afternoon and take off for parts unknown for a picnic, a hike, or a day of cross-country skiing. Life seemed more of an adventure than a struggle. What happened?

"Things have to change," she says. "There's more to life than dreaming of a nap."

In a burst of sleep-deprived inspiration, she draws up a list: Carolyn's Bill of Rights.

1. I have the right to 8 solid hours of sleep a night.
2. I have the right to turn off my cell phone and beeper at a reasonable hour.
3. I have the right to go "off-duty" to spend some time on *me*.
4. I have the right to ask my husband to help more with the kids and Mom.

5. I have the right to live a healthier life—in the foods I eat, the vitamins I take, and the exercises I do.

6. I have the right to play—with my husband, with my kids, on my own.

Carolyn has reached her breaking point. How about you?

Come on. Tag along with Carolyn. Join her on a journey from energy bust to boom. By the end of this book, you, too, will know how to fight female fatigue syndrome.

If Carolyn can do it, so can you.

This Thing Called Energy

It's 6 A.M., and the sun is just peeking through the blinds in Carolyn's bedroom. She's still asleep, but her brain is already at work, signaling changes in critical chemicals and hormones throughout her body that serve as an internal alarm clock. By the time the buzzer blasts on the alarm beside the bed, her body temperature has begun to rise, and tiny photoreceptors in her eyes have begun to signal a gland in her brain to slow its secretion of what some may call the sleep hormone, melatonin.

It's time to wake up.

But it takes a hot shower and three cups of coffee before her grogginess disappears. For the rest of the morning, Carolyn is on a roll—typing reports, tackling those toppling piles of paper, and planning her boss's business trip. Until 2 P.M. Suddenly, her eyes seem to have gained 10 pounds, and she has typed the same sentence over and over. She struggles through and finds her second wind around 4 P.M., a blast that stays with her through the evening until she conks out at 11.

Energy peaks and valleys like Carolyn's are endemic. Some are our own doing, caused by late nights, caffeinated pick-me-ups, or heavy meals. But the conductor behind our energy levels resides deep in our brains. A complex clump of cells directs the symphony of daily hormone releases, body temperature changes, and blood pressure shifts called circadian rhythms. Oddly, our circadian rhythms run on a 25-hour cycle, which doesn't match Earth's 24-hour day. So every day, we are forced to reset our natural, 25-hour body clock, which is perhaps one more reason we're all so tired.

It's important to understand the physical rhythms that guide our days so we can learn to maximize our peaks and plan for our valleys.

Live without Time

For 2 weeks, Lynne Lamberg, a medical writer from Baltimore, lived without time. "There were no clocks, no radios, no televisions, no windows, and no indications of time from the researchers with whom I interacted," says Lamberg, coauthor of *The Body Clock Guide to Better Health: How to Use Your Body's Natural Clock to Fight Illness and Achieve Maximum Health.* When she wanted to go to sleep, researchers shut down the lights; they turned them on again only when she told them she was ready to get up. Using volunteers like Lamberg, scientists hope to discover what happens to our body clocks when they're allowed to run on their own, natural schedule.

Lamberg spent her timeless days writing, reading, riding an exercise bike, listening to music, and taking tests to measure her alertness and mental abilities. She ate three meals a day. "One day they asked me to stay up as late as I could," she remembers. Later, she learned she had managed to stay awake for nearly 23 hours and slept for about 7.5 hours, stretching her days to about 30 hours.

When she wasn't trying to break records for staying awake, Lamberg felt good in the lab. "I slept quite well, I was healthy, and I had as much, if not more, energy as usual. I just followed my biological clock." And her clock ran free on a 25-hour schedule.

Once she reviewed the results of the study, Lamberg's attitude toward sleep changed. "In the lab, you sleep as long as you want, so I thought I was sleeping 9 to 10 hours instead of my usual 7," she says. "But I was surprised to learn that I slept only 7 to 7¾ hours each night, which is my internally determined amount of necessary sleep." Before the time lab, she woke every day to the alarm clock feeling groggy and tired. "Now I don't pay attention to clocks," she says. "I just leave the blinds open and let light awaken me, and I always wake up at about the same time, even though my bedtime may vary an hour or so from night to night."

The Power of Light

There's a lesson to be learned in Lamberg's experience. Light drives energy. It works like this.

On various parts of your body—your eyes, the backs of your knees, and possibly other places—are nerve endings, called photoreceptors, that absorb light. Once those photoreceptors pick up the light, they send a signal to the pineal gland in the brain to stop producing melatonin, the so-called sleep hormone. Scientists suspect that when it's dark, and melatonin is secreted, the hormone signals your body temperature to drop, which is ideal for rest. With light comes a cessation of melatonin secretion and a gradually increasing body temperature, which is ideal for alertness.

Your temperature hits its low point at 4 A.M. Then, during the last hours of sleep, your temperature rises, helping you to rise along with it. These aren't huge fluctuations—just 3 to 4 degrees—but they're enough to signal your body.

Beat the Clock

Wonder why you're so tired after we switch to daylight saving time in the spring? Because you're asked to wake up an hour earlier than usual. This can be difficult, especially for night owls. Your body knows it's only 6 A.M., even though the clock says 7.

Within a few days, however, your body clock should reset itself to match your watch. If not, you could be sleep-deprived or have a sleep disorder, so check with your doctor. To help your internal hands adjust, the National Sleep Foundation recommends the following steps.

- On the night before the time change, get at least 8 hours of sleep.
- Go to bed at your regular time on Saturday, but get up a half-hour earlier on Sunday morning. Most important, make sure you see the sunlight when you wake up. (In the fall, delay bedtime by a half-hour on Saturday night, and go to bed at your regular time on Sunday.)
- Take a nap on Sunday before 4 P.M.
- Get 8 hours of sleep Sunday night.

Experts consulted: Margaret Moline, Ph.D., director of the Sleep–Wake Disorders Center, New York Presbyterian Hospital, New York City, and Charmane Eastman, Ph.D., director of the Biological Rhythms Research Lab, Rush–Presbyterian–St. Luke's Medical Center, Chicago

That's why melatonin is often taken as a supplement to help with jet lag and sleep problems. The long-term effects of supplemental melatonin have not been thoroughly studied, however, so it should be taken only under the supervision of a doctor; supplemental melatonin has many possible side effects.

Body temperature continues to fluctuate throughout the day. It rises during the mid- to late morning, which is one reason we often feel so energized during this time. In early afternoon, it dips slightly—perhaps contributing to that post-lunch slump. Then it rises again in the mid- to late afternoon. This may account for the "second wind" we get around 4 P.M. By 11, we've turned the lights out, melatonin production has already started, and our temperatures fall in preparation for sleep. At the same time, our heart rates and blood pressures drop in accordance with our bodies' natural rhythms.

The World around You

Beyond your own biochemical brew are external cues that foul your circadian pacemakers. These cues keep you on the 24-hour, circadian schedule rather than the 25-hour timetable your body wants to embrace.

Here are suggestions to moderate the cues experts have identified.

Smooth out erratic routines. "If your schedule is irregular, you can give yourself a kind of jet lag without leaving home," says Margaret Moline, Ph.D., director of the Sleep–Wake Disorders Center at New York Presbyterian Hospital in New York City. The 25 million Americans who work graveyard or split shifts know this very well.

Because they sleep when the rest of the world is awake, night-shift workers experience more interruptions to their sleep, such as noise, sunlight, and higher room temperature.

So they are chronically sleep-deprived. Since sleep helps rejuvenate your organ systems and your brain so that they function properly, this chronic lack of sleep jeopardizes health, on-the-job safety, memory, mood, and performance. Consequently, shift workers are at risk for concentration problems, weight gain, heart problems, and more colds and flu bouts.

To beat the problems inherent in shift work, try the following measures.

- Begin adjusting to a new work schedule several days before it starts. Maybe you changed jobs and now have to get up 2 hours earlier to commute to work. To adjust, go to bed and wake up 15 minutes earlier each day in the week prior to your actual first day, suggests Dr. Moline.
- Wind down before bed by taking a warm bath, lowering the room temperature in your bedroom, and avoiding such brain-activating activities as balancing your checkbook and watching a suspenseful movie.
- If work ends during daylight, wear dark glasses on the ride home to prevent your body from going into daytime mode. At home, darken your bedroom and bathroom with light-blocking curtains and wear eye shades while you sleep.
- Soundproof your surroundings by unplugging the phone, wearing earplugs, and using a white noise machine, such as a fan.

Say good night to Letterman. Your ancestors knew when to go to sleep and wake up. But today the boundaries between night and day have largely disappeared. Most of us need an average of 8 to 8½ hours of sleep a night, but we get only an average of 6 hours and 41 minutes.

"Adequate sleep is the amount you need to be alert and functioning during the day," says Dr. Moline. "But if you
(continued on page 22)

Are You a Lark or an Owl?

Morning people are larks, and evening people are owls. Owls tend to select later bedtimes and get up later than larks, and they tend to have a harder time adapting to social demands because much of the rest of the world rises and sets with the sun.

Energy-wise, larks feel more vigilant in the earlier part of the day, while owls reach their peak in alertness later. Scientists don't know for sure why people are larks or owls, or how they become that way. Some think it may relate to the time of year we're born. A study at the University of Bologna in Italy showed that more morning people are born in autumn and winter, and more evening people are born in spring and summer.

To assess whether you are a lark or an owl, take this short quiz.

1. If you had no obligations, what time would you choose to go to bed?
   a. Before 10:30 P.M.
   b. Between 10:30 and midnight
   c. After midnight

2. With no obligations, what time would you get up?
   a. Before 7 A.M.
   b. Between 7 and 9 A.M.
   c. After 9 A.M.

3. An hour before you go to bed during the workweek, how sleepy do you feel?
   a. I feel pretty okay.
   b. It depends on the day.
   c. Exhausted

4. A friend has asked you to exercise with her a few times a week. She suggests hitting the track from 7 to 8 A.M. How do you react?
   a. Ugh. There's no way.
   b. I think I'll be okay.
   c. No problem—morning's my favorite time to work out.

5. How alert do you feel in the first half-hour you're awake?
   a. Not alert—sleepy
   b. Depends on the day
   c. Alert and refreshed

6. In the morning, how much do you rely on caffeine to get you going?
   a. I'm a zombie without it; I drink it all morning.
   b. I drink it some days.
   c. I don't rely on caffeine at all.

Scoring

1. a–0; b–2; c–4
2. a–0; b–2; c–4
3. a–4; b–2; c–0
4. a–4; b–2; c–0
5. a–4; b–2; c–0
6. a–4; b–2; c–0

0–5: You're a lark.
6–10: You have more lark than owl tendencies.
11–15: You aren't really either.
16–20: You have more owl tendencies.
21–24: You're an owl.

go to sleep late and wake up early, your brain may still want to be sleeping." That's why you feel groggy even after your third cup of coffee. Further, even 8 hours of sleep is no guarantee of energy. Just two 15-minute disruptions, by either your child or your partner's snoring, can affect your energy level the next day, she says.

To get a good night's sleep, experts offer the following tips.

- Relieve some stress before bed by doing something that relaxes you, such as talking to a trusted friend on the phone or meditating.
- A troubling thought at 3 A.M. can be a major sleep interruption. Set aside time in the day to think about situations that are bothering you and how to remedy them.
- Alcohol at bedtime may help induce sleep at first, but it will disrupt your rest later in the night by awakening you or giving you nightmares, and it may leave you with a headache in the morning.

Beat the seasons. Lack of sunlight in the winter may lead to seasonal affective disorder (SAD), a form of depression in which you feel sad only during certain months of the year. Scientists suspect it has to do with a disruption of our circadian rhythms. Long winter nights may cause us to secrete more melatonin. The hormone's sedating effects may render us depressed. If you have had less energy and have felt anxious and depressed for 2 consecutive winter months, you may be suffering from SAD and should talk to your doctor. She is likely to suggest light therapy, which involves exposure to special lamps that are 10 to 20 times brighter than normal indoor lights.

Treat weekends like workdays. You can't treat yourself to a noon wake-up on the weekends and then expect to joyfully leap out of bed at 6:30 Monday morning. The price you pay is Sunday insomnia—when you lie in bed, wide awake, at your normal 11 P.M. bedtime. To keep your rhythms balanced, wake up at the same time every day, even on the weekends.

Put safety first. Each year, driver drowsiness causes about 56,000 automobile crashes, killing more than 1,550 people. Half of us admit we drive while drowsy. And nearly 17 percent of us have actually fallen asleep at the wheel.

To avoid becoming one of these statistics, experts recommend the following preventive measures.

- Take a 15- to 20-minute nap before driving if you are too sleepy to drive safely. Even a small dose of sleep will make you more refreshed and capable of driving.
- Bring a talkative passenger. Conversation is a great eye-opener.
- Be extra careful when driving between 2 A.M. and 6 A.M., when your circadian rhythms are in sleep mode—or avoid driving at these times altogether.
- Recognize the warning signs of driving fatigue: eyes closing or going out of focus, thoughts wandering, or your car drifting off the road. If you experience drowsiness, you should not be behind the wheel.

Adjust to Your Own Clock

You don't have to be a victim to your rhythms. There are ways you can control them, instead of allowing them to control you.

Keep an energy diary. "Be aware of your own patterns and when you function best," recommends Cheryl Dellasega, Ph.D., associate director of research in general internal medicine at Pennsylvania State University's Hershey Medical Center. For one day, set the alarm on your watch or pager to go off every hour; then write in your "energy diary" how you feel at that particular time.

Measure your rhythms. Take your oral temperature every hour from the time you wake up in the morning to the time you go to bed. (Don't exercise on that day, and avoid eating or drinking right before taking your temperature; both activities raise body temperature.) Then map the temperatures on graph paper or a spreadsheet. Plot your temperature on the vertical axis and the time of day on the horizontal axis. You may see peaks during the high-energy times you noted in your diary and valleys during your low-energy times.

Once you've mapped your downtimes, you can change the way you react to those rhythms. If you know you dip after lunch, for instance, don't schedule intense work during that time, or else build a 15-minute nap into your daily calendar.

Exhaustion Only a Woman Could Know

Carolyn bolts awake, her sheets soaked with sweat. She peeks at the alarm clock, only to find its red numbers glaring 3:12 A.M. Not again! She scrambles out of bed and staggers down the stairs for a glass of ice water. As she rounds the corner, she's startled to see Jocelyn at the table, her head propped on her hand.

"What's the matter?" Carolyn asks as she holds an ice cube against her steaming skin.

"Can't sleep, Mom." Then the girl glances at her mother. "Why are you all sweaty?"

"Hot flashes. You'll know in 30 years or so. Why can't *you* sleep?"

"I dunno. I usually sleep like a rock. Come to think of it, I've had trouble sleeping a couple times these past few months, and you know, it's always been during my period."

"Really? I wonder what that's all about," says Carolyn as she warms some milk for her daughter on the stove.

Jocelyn sips the warm milk while she and her mother talk about their dreams. They connect. And something good comes of a sleepless night.

Hormones: A Culprit behind Female Fatigue

As Carolyn and Jocelyn have discovered, some of our exhaustion—and disturbed sleep—comes from the very things that make us women. Our hormones.

Hormones do more than prime us for pregnancy and strengthen our bones. They mold us into who we are. They give us our feminine curves, our supple skin, and our high-pitched giggles.

The challenge is keeping our hormones in check. When they're balanced, we feel energized. But they naturally have more peaks and valleys than the Swiss Alps—and can leave us feeling like we just *climbed* the Alps. Fortunately, there are ways to recognize those high and low points and steps you can take to minimize the energy-sapping valleys.

That Time of the Month

It has been about 20 days since your last period, and you're so sluggish you feel like you're moving in slow motion.

"Most women complain about fatigue the day or so before their periods and the first day or two of their periods," says Ricki Pollycove, M.D., an obstetrician/gynecologist and director of patient education at the California Pacific Medical Center Breast Health Center in San Francisco. We're tired then because of dropping levels of estrogen and progesterone, which affect various other hormones and body systems and processes, including the following:

Serotonin. This brain chemical/hormone is involved in sleep, mood, pain, and appetite. Higher levels of serotonin increase the amount of deep sleep we get each night and improve our overall well-being. And higher levels of estrogen support higher levels of serotonin. So when estrogen levels drop, so, too, does the amount of serotonin in our brains. One way to boost serotonin levels is with vigorous physical exercise, says Dr. Pollycove.

Metabolism. Some women require higher levels of estrogen to keep their metabolisms working at peak efficiency. Since metabolism is what turns food into fuel, if it's running at half speed, so are we. During our periods, when estrogen levels drop, we're dragging. To find out if you have low estrogen levels, ask your doctor about a saliva test that can be used to measure your hormone levels, Dr. Pollycove suggests.

Stress hormones. There's a synergistic effect between estrogen and stress hormones such as cortisol and adrenaline. The more stress we're under, the more stress hormones we release, which seems to plunge our estrogen levels even lower—all the more reason to pencil in a massage just before your period starts.

Sleep. Progesterone's role in a woman's cycle is to prepare her uterus for pregnancy. But if she's not pregnant, progesterone levels drop just before her period, sending a signal to slough off the blood-rich lining of her uterus. In the years right before menopause, when our ovaries slow down their progesterone production, sleep disturbances plague us even more. For some women, using a progesterone supplement just before their periods start may help, says Dr. Pollycove. It may, however, result in increased water retention, she says.

You might try applying a progesterone cream, available at health food stores, before hitting the sack, suggests Dr. Pollycove. For best results, apply the cream to your abdomen or the inner parts of your arms or thighs. Use the cream every night for the last 10 days of your cycle. (Day 1 of your approximately 28-day cycle is your first day of bleeding.) Or ask your doctor about a progesterone pill such as Prometrium. This prescription drug works much

What Does "Tired" Mean?

Fatigue is such a broad term that it's almost useless in diagnosing a condition, says Dianne Delva, M.D., associate professor of family medicine at Queen's University in Kingston, Ontario.

Lab tests aren't much better: One study showed that fewer than 10 percent of laboratory tests for fatigue helped determine a diagnosis. A better method is plain old *talking*.

Asking specific questions about how fatigue affects your life is the most effective way for your doctor to uncover the problem, says Dr. Delva. Often no medical treatment is needed, just minor adjustments in sleeping, eating, exercising, or working habits. In fact, almost half of women who say they're fatigued are actually depressed.

One objective indicator of fatigue is its relation to time. It's either acute, prolonged, or chronic. Acute fatigue lasts

the same as the cream. Your doctor may want to measure your progesterone levels first before prescribing progesterone supplements, notes Dr. Pollycove.

Moving into Menopause

The hot flashes so prevalent as we approach menopause result from dropping estrogen levels. During a hot flash, blood rushes to the surface of your skin until you feel like you're standing in a furnace. You sweat, and your breathing and heart rate speed up. Experts speculate we get hot flashes because the climate control center in the brain reads the perimenopausal drop in estrogen as a drop in body temperature and tries to warm things up to compensate.

less than 1 month, and the cause is often obvious, such as the flu or the first trimester of pregnancy.

Prolonged fatigue typically lasts between 1 and 6 months. Many women who are depressed have prolonged fatigue. Hypothyroidism, in which the thyroid doesn't produce enough of its hormone, can also result in low energy levels. If you don't seek help for these conditions, you may stray into chronic fatigue territory—more than 6 months of exhaustion. Don't try to cope with chronic fatigue on your own, cautions Dr. Delva, since it could reflect a serious health concern such as type 2 diabetes.

Be specific, says Dr. Delva. If you're not sure what's making you tired, tell your doctor these things: what you are doing when you are tired; when during the day or month you are most tired; how long it has been like this; why you think you feel this way; and how, exactly, being "tired" feels.

Flashes (or baby boomer power surges, as some women call them) are especially prevalent at night because the part of the body that "turns on" a hot flash is sensitive to levels of estrogen, sugar, and alcohol, all of which drop while we sleep, Dr. Pollycove explains.

One solution (other than not drinking before bed) may be low-dose birth control pills, which contain about one-fifth to one-third the amount of estrogen found in traditional birth control pills, says Dr. Pollycove. They've been found to help with hot flashes, sleep disturbances, fatigue, and PMS symptoms.

Another reason for sleep disturbances as you enter menopause has to do with the male hormone testosterone. Just as men's bodies produce estrogen, your body produces small amounts of testosterone. Because your body makes such a tiny amount of the hormone, you're very sensitive to any fluctuations. Just a slight drop in testosterone can disrupt your normal rate of metabolism and leave you feeling drained, not to mention less than interested in sex.

Your ovaries make about one-third of your testosterone. So if a woman has a hysterectomy and has her ovaries removed, she will experience a sudden drop not only in estrogen but also in testosterone. Many doctors don't know this, so they fail to warn their patients. If you've had this operation and noticed a corresponding decline in sex drive and energy, ask to have your testosterone levels tested.

Natural menopause, however, may eventually have much the same effect. That's what happened to Susan Rako, M.D., a Boston psychiatrist who in 1996 brought the often overlooked problem of testosterone deficiency to the forefront with her book *The Hormone of Desire: The Truth about Testosterone, Sexuality, and Menopause.* She discovered that she had low levels of not only estrogen but also testosterone. Her symptoms appeared gradually over a period of 3 to 4 months. As for her energy level, she says that she felt "flat." "It affected everything," she remembers.

No wonder. Tests showed she had almost no testosterone in her system.

Dr. Rako was 47 at the time and going through perimenopause, the several years of irregular periods that most women experience before periods totally cease. During these transition years, our ovaries produce not only less estrogen but also less testosterone. The adrenal glands, the other significant source of testosterone, also produce less of it as we age.

Further, if you choose estrogen or hormone replacement therapy for menopausal symptoms, the treatment actually *decreases* the level of usable testosterone in your body. That's because estrogen boosts levels of globulin—a substance that binds to and inactivates some of the testosterone—thereby keeping in our bodies a pool of testosterone that we can't use. Thus, the more estrogen, the less usable testosterone.

A study at Baylor College of Medicine in Houston found that giving estrogen replacement therapy to 28 postmenopausal women for 12 weeks caused their testosterone levels to drop 42 percent. On the other hand, several other studies show that women treated with supplemental estrogen and testosterone have greater energy and a better sense of well-being than those treated with estrogen alone. In the past, doctors were reluctant to give women supplemental testosterone because too much could make them feel irritable and anxious, cause them to develop facial hair and acne, and increase their risk of developing diabetes and high cholesterol.

Today, more doctors test and treat women for testosterone deficiency, says Barbara Sherwin, Ph.D., professor of psychology, obstetrics, and gynecology at McGill University in Montreal, Quebec. If you suspect a testosterone deficiency is to blame for your fatigue and low libido, find a doctor who's willing to test your hormone levels and, if necessary, treat you with supplemental testosterone.

The Butterfly in Your Throat

Just below your Adam's apple sits a butterfly-shaped gland, the thyroid. Call it the energy gland. It produces hormones that have a hand in nearly every body system, affecting everything from your heart rate and body temperature to how fast you metabolize food.

A thyroid that doesn't pump out enough hormones is a common (and often overlooked) cause of fatigue—so common, in fact, that as many as 10 percent of all women may have some degree of thyroid deficiency. In fact, women make up the vast majority of the 11 million Americans with hypothyroidism, meaning an underactive thyroid.

Because of the gland's far-reaching effects throughout the body, an underactive thyroid can cause a slew of symptoms, such as fatigue, depression, constipation, dry skin, hair loss, hoarseness, cold sensitivity, muscle or joint aches, and increased menstrual flow.

One of the critical areas affected by a decrease in thyroid hormones is metabolism. So while that extra scoop of ice cream and those couch potato habits may indeed be the cause of the extra 20 pounds you're carrying, so could an underactive thyroid. Typically, the hormone "turns on" adrenaline-like parts of cells that speed up the rate at which we turn food into energy. Too little output means it's that much harder for your cells to burn the fuel they need for energy. Ergo, fatigue and weight gain.

The most common cause of an underactive thyroid is autoimmune hypothyroidism, sometimes called Hashimoto's thyroiditis or Hashimoto's disease, after the Japanese doctor who first described the disorder. The immune systems of women with this condition attack and damage their own thyroid glands, leaving them unable to pump out enough hormones. Autoimmune hypothyroidism tends to run in families, so it's best to know your family history.

An underactive thyroid is also common in women who've had radioactive iodine to treat an *overactive* thyroid or those who've had radiation to treat head or neck cancers.

Yet another reason women are more susceptible to having underactive thyroids is—you guessed it—an imbalance in female hormones. If your estrogen levels are high compared with your progesterone levels, it can throw off your thyroid hormone levels, says Mark Stengler, N.D., director of natural medicine at Personal Physicians clinic in La Jolla, California, associate clinical professor at the

National College of Naturopathic Medicine in Portland, Oregon, and author of *The Natural Physician*. Called estrogen dominance, this condition occurs when there is not enough progesterone to balance the effects of estrogen. High estrogen levels suppress thyroid stimulating hormone (TSH), a messenger hormone sent from the brain to tell the thyroid to make thyroid hormone. If the message can't get through, the thyroid hormone doesn't get produced.

Women are also more at risk for hypothyroidism simply because we tend to live longer than men. As with many body systems, the older we get, the less effectively our thyroids work.

Usually, all it takes to diagnose this condition is a simple $25 blood test called a thyroid stimulating hormone test. Don't put it off. Hypothyroidism that goes undiagnosed for too long can lead to high cholesterol and increase your risk of heart disease. That's one reason the American Thyroid Association recommends that all women age 35 and older have a routine thyroid test every 5 years.

Treatment is also simple: taking synthetic thyroid hormones, perhaps for the rest of your life. Once your doctor determines the right dose, you'll have to get your thyroid hormone levels rechecked only about once a year.

The Hormone before the Hormone

Erase wrinkles! Live longer! Boost your sex drive! Fight disease!

That's the promise for the "miracle" hormone, the fountain of youth, DHEA. Short for dehydroepiandrosterone, DHEA is a precursor to testosterone and estrogen. If DHEA levels are low, testosterone levels may also be low. Preliminary research is now being conducted to determine what role, if any, DHEA levels play in predicting fatigue, low sex drive, and mood problems.

Older Women Don't Need Less Sleep

You need the same amount of sleep at any age—about 8½ hours. In fact, your average total sleep time increases slightly after age 65. Instead of sleeping all your hours in one nighttime block, you may take daytime naps. But daytime drowsiness is not an inevitable result of aging. And naps can interfere with your ability to sleep at night. When you feel sleepy, try going for a walk, gardening, or doing other outdoor activities.

As we age, many things interfere with our ability to get all our sleep at one time. Our sleep–wake rhythms become less distinct. We suffer from bladder problems. We may experience arthritis, osteoporosis, heart disease, heartburn, or any number of medical maladies that affect the quality of our sleep. And many medicines can cause either drowsiness or sleeplessness. If you think your sleeping problem may be associated with your medication, discuss it with your doctor.

"DHEA and testosterone levels go hand in hand," says Arthur Schwartz, Ph.D., researcher and microbiologist at Temple University Medical School in Philadelphia, who has been studying DHEA for 25 years. You can, in fact, have a decline in testosterone levels and still have normal DHEA levels. So even if your ovaries are producing less testosterone—because you are on the Pill, are undergoing menopause, or have just had a hysterectomy—your levels of DHEA, produced predominantly by the adrenal gland, would remain unchanged.

Your DHEA levels are highest when you're in your twenties; as you age, your adrenal glands produce less DHEA. By the time you hit your seventies and eighties, the glands produce only 30 percent of what they made when you were younger.

Another problem may be advanced sleep phase syndrome. That's when you nod off in front of the 6 P.M. news but arise before sunup. While there's a tendency for this to develop as we age, you're not doomed to this fate. Your best course of action is to spend time in the daylight between 4 and 6 P.M., keep bright lights on once it gets dark, and try to stay up a little later than normal. Then go to sleep in a pitch-black bedroom. This marked difference in light and darkness sends a signal through your optic nerve to your brain that it's time to produce the sleep hormone melatonin.

Another reason for sleep problems as you age is lack of activity. So get plenty of exercise during the day.

Expert consulted: Donna Arand, Ph.D., clinical director, Sleep Disorders Center of Kettering Medical Center, Kettering, Ohio

The key to curbing this DHEA decline is to keep your adrenal glands healthy, says Ray Sahelian, M.D., a physician in Marina del Rey, California, and author of *Mind Boosters: A Guide to Natural Supplements That Enhance Your Mind, Memory, and Mood*. That means adopting a healthy, active lifestyle. No surprises here: Exercise regularly; eat a balanced, low-fat diet with adequate omega-3 fatty acids (found in cold-water fish like tuna, salmon, and mackerel); get enough sleep; and learn ways to reduce stress.

If you do have unexplained fatigue, bad moods, and a low sex drive, ask your doctor to check your DHEA levels. If they're low, talk to her about DHEA supplements. In one German study, 24 women whose adrenal glands didn't produce normal amounts of DHEA reported feeling more energetic and less depressed after taking 50 milligrams of DHEA for 4 months.

But don't self-supplement with DHEA. "It's a double-edged sword," Dr. Sahelian says. "DHEA and other hormones available over the counter have benefits, but they can do harm if misused." They can cause irritability, acne, thinning hair, and menstrual cycle changes. "These are all signs you're taking too much or don't need to be taking it at all," he says.

And because we convert DHEA into other hormones, Dr. Sahelian adds, supplementing with DHEA may increase the risk of breast and other reproductive cancers.

PART TWO

Energy Drainers

How Little Things
Can Wear You Down

It's Friday morning, and Carolyn is zipping down the road of life. Well, the one to her office, anyway.

She's doing her usual 65-mile-an-hour clip, thankful it's the end of the week. Hopefully, she can recuperate this weekend from her frenetic pace. But first she has to get through today.

She starts ticking off her to-do list in her mind. That gift to buy for her cousin's wedding. Hitting the grocery store to get supplies for the homemade cookies she promised Jocelyn. A pile of work to plow through. But she has one nice thing to look forward to: dinner out Saturday with Ben's coworker and his wife.

Suddenly, she notices flashes of yellow ahead and a plethora of blinking red brake lights. The cars in front of her begin to slow. To crawl. To stop.

Not another morning tie-up! She just does *not* have time for this. But she's nowhere near an exit. She's stuck, with her heart pounding and a torrent of worries shooting through her like lightning bolts.

Five minutes, then 10. Half an hour later, the cars

ahead begin moving. By then, however, Carolyn is a wreck. Her car didn't overheat, but she sure did. She's fuming, frustrated, and emotionally and physically spent before she even pulls into the office parking lot.

Studies show that it's not the major life events like losing your job or getting married that most emotionally exhaust us but those annoying everyday occurrences like car trouble or running late for work. "Those chronic little stressors are the ones that really can do damage, particularly if we don't realize what's going on," says Angela Stroup, R.N., a certified hypnotherapist, mentor/coach, and adjunct assistant professor of family and community medicine at Eastern Virginia Medical School in Norfolk.

Over time, the blips pile up like those cars on the highway, chronically deflating your vigor, both physically and emotionally, says Ruth E. Quillian, Ph.D., a health psychologist at Duke University's Center for Living in Durham, North Carolina. They wear on your psyche, weaken your immunity to colds and other illnesses, raise your blood pressure, and even set you up for heart disease, the leading cause of death in women. One reason: These life stressors often make people angry, and inappropriately expressed anger is physically and emotionally draining. It taxes your health and vitality but doesn't solve the problem. One study suggests the angrier you are, the greater your risk for heart problems. This is particularly true for unresolved anger, says Dr. Quillian.

Like our ancestors of 10,000 years ago, we're still programmed for the fight-or-flight response, Dr. Quillian explains. When we sense a threat or obstacle, our bodies produce adrenaline, raising our blood sugar and preparing us for action.

If you're fighting tigers, that's useful. But if you're sitting in a car on a highway to nowhere, that adrenaline rush is doing battle with you instead.

"If it happens over and over, you have an energy drain," says Dr. Quillian.

There are better ways to deal with life's annoyances. You can learn not only to cope with the express lines that aren't, the surly clerks, and the just-bought milk that's already spoiled, but also to flourish, turning those stressors to our advantage and reaping renewed vigor where chaos once reigned. It's a trait worth learning, not only for today but for tomorrow. One study conducted by the prestigious Mayo Clinic suggests that people who face challenges with optimism live longer, healthier lives than pessimists.

Remember the Serenity Prayer

The Serenity Prayer goes like this: God, grant me the serenity to accept the things I cannot change, the courage to change the things I can, and the wisdom to know the difference. That's a good philosophy to apply throughout your life, suggests Dr. Quillian.

"Expect the craziness of the world and learn to find the humor in it," she urges. "Do yourself a favor by not exhausting your emotional energies on situations you can't control."

And stop expecting perfection. We know *we* can't do everything perfectly, so why should we expect anyone else to? "We have become pretty extreme in our expectations," Dr. Quillian says.

These high expectations took root in the late 1960s as more women began working outside the home. No longer did we have one person earning the dollars and one person performing the "home work." So we grew to rely on others to do many of those services for us. As a result, service industries proliferated: We pay people to do our laundry, gardening, and vacuuming and to deliver our dinners, take care of our kids, and wash our cars.

"The lack of time is a stress factor, but we have added to that the lack of face-to-face relationships," says Deborah Cowles, Ph.D., associate professor of marketing at Virginia Commonwealth University in Richmond. Plus, many of us work in service industries ourselves—nursing, selling, catering. We're already dealing all day long with people we don't know.

Add to that a widespread labor shortage that makes good employees hard to find, especially at minimum wage. The result? You can wind up with an exhaustive cycle of raised expectations, too little time, and inevitable disappointments.

You can save yourself some headaches—and energy—by learning to expect and plan for interruptions, errors, missed connections. Here are three specific suggestions.

Plan for delays. When you need to run an errand, try to give yourself a little extra time—say, 30 minutes instead of 15 to get the groceries. Then you won't be so dependent on a flawless string of service, Dr. Cowles says.

Be empathetic. Put yourself in the other person's shoes. Research shows that when we react with empathy, we stimulate the release of feel-good hormones called endorphins. Also, we build a social support system—one of the strongest protectors of our emotional and physical well-being—even when we just say hello to that cashier we see each week. "It's a skill that has to be practiced," admits Dr. Quillian. But it may be worth it.

Laugh. Studies of women executives show that those with a healthy sense of humor feel less stressed and have a higher sense of self-esteem than their less jovial peers. Even just smiling results in a release of endorphins to soothe our psyches.

This doesn't mean you should routinely accept poor service. That's a pattern that can erode self-esteem and

Instant Vacation

Boost your energy with 3-minute "mini-vacations," suggests psychotherapist Edie Raether, of Raleigh, North Carolina. Mentally experience some relaxing spot, such as a mountain valley or a beautiful beach. "Pick your peacefulness and go with it." This visualization "puts the process of relaxation into your body," she says. Afterward, you'll have more energy.

energy. While it may be initially taxing to learn how, taking appropriate action relieves stress and is invigorating, says Dr. Quillian. For specific tips on what you can do to improve the service you receive, see page 47.

On the Road Again

With more people on the road than ever before, highway logjams are almost a way of life, especially if you commute into a large city for work.

If you have an "Oh, no, not this" reaction when you run into traffic jams, you've just given a powerful jump start to the stress/tension cycle that will drain your energy, says Judith Kessler, Psy.D., a behavioral psychologist and adjunct instructor at the National College for Naturopathic Medicine in Portland, Oregon. The key is to reframe the situation so that it actually brings new energy to your day, she says.

How do you do that? Go with the flow—or nonflow, says Dr. Quillian.

First, if you have a cellular phone, use it to let people know you'll be late.

Next? Breathe!

When we're stressed, we tend to hold our breath or breathe less deeply, says Stroup. Our muscles tighten, our heart rate quickens, our blood pressure rises, and our pupils dilate.

"The most useful tool you have is your breath," Dr. Quillian says. Breathing deeply, from your abdomen, makes it almost impossible to stay stressed.

As you breathe deeply, you are calmed and energized. Your heart rate slows, your blood pressure is coaxed downward, and your brain halts the production of stress hormones and jump-starts your parasympathetic nervous system, which is associated with rest and healing. Blood vessels relax, circulation improves, your pulse slows.

You're telling your body: "False alarm. This is not a tiger."

A traffic jam is one of the best places to practice deep breathing, Dr. Kessler says.

The next time you're stuck behind the wheel, practice what Stroup calls "the three Rs breath." First, take a deep breath through your nose and think of the word *relax*. Then pause for 1 to 2 seconds and think of the word *rest*. Finally, exhale through your mouth and "release" all of the tensions of the day. Make sure your exhalation is twice as long as your inhalation, she says.

Do this several times as you imagine a pleasant memory or place. Drift to a placid lakeside or wooded mountaintop. You don't even have to close your eyes for your mind to take the clue.

Our brains are so smart yet so dumb, says Barbara Bailey Reinhold, Ed.D., director of the career development office at Smith College in Northampton, Massachusetts, and author of *Toxic Work: How to Overcome Stress, Overload, and Burnout and Revitalize Your Career.* "They believe what we tell them."

Accept the traffic jam as an opportunity, Dr. Kessler suggests. How often do you get quiet time alone? Enjoy the peace, the solitude. Revel in it. Feel your body. Tense, and then relax, your toes, ankles, fists, shoulders. Try to stay in the moment, instead of fast-forwarding to the day's obligations or worries.

Other tactics?

- Keep a book or reading for work in the car to peruse if traffic is at a standstill.
- Carry a notepad to write letters or make a shopping list.
- Stash an empty grocery bag under the seat so you can clean out that messy glove compartment or the console between the driver's and passenger's seats.
- Listen to tapes or CDs that are inspirational or invigorating, by Billy Graham, the Bee Gees, or Beethoven. One survey by the marketing research and consulting firm Roper Starch Worldwide showed that more than half of us call music our top stress buster.

How to Handle Poor Service

It's lunch hour, and Carolyn zips into the department store parking lot exactly 12 minutes after leaving her office. Hmmm. That leaves about 30 minutes to sleuth out a wedding gift for her cousin, pay, and run, if she hopes to gulp down any lunch at all.

She hustles toward housewares, where she quickly settles on a lovely floral serving platter. At the checkout, she picks the shortest line: only two people ahead of her. She checks her watch; she has several minutes to spare, even if the cashier *is* moving about as slowly as a turtle on a country road.

Finally, it's her turn. The cashier runs the platter over the scanner. *Beep.* Again she tries to scan it. *Beep.*

"Do you know the price on this?" the cashier calls to another employee several lanes away.

"No, but I'll go check. Where'd she find it?"

"I'm sure it costs $39.99," says Carolyn, growing impatient. The cashier ignores her. Two minutes. Five minutes. Finally the other clerk returns.

"Thirty-nine ninety-nine."

Carolyn is furious and feels like hurling the platter to the floor, along with the cashier. Instead, she grits her teeth, hands the cashier a $100 bill, and stomps out to the car, her change crunched in her fist.

Once there, she stuffs the money in her wallet, then pulls it back out. There's a little more than $30. But she should have more than $50 in change.

She has neither the time nor the energy for this. Angry with herself, the store, the cashier, and her cousin for getting married in the first place, she drives off, tires squealing. Then she spends the rest of the afternoon fuming about the incident and beating herself up for not going back to the store—thus scoring a big fat zero on the energy scorecard.

Like Carolyn, we often don't know how to express anger, how to verbalize what bothers us, Dr. Kessler says. That in itself is an energy pillager.

But we reenergize and relieve our stress by taking calm, appropriate action, Dr. Cowles says. If you're frustrated with the service, go back and talk to the cashier or the store manager. It's your job as a consumer to speak up when you're dissatisfied with a service or product, she says. Most businesses want to know if you're unhappy. It's a competitive world out there; they need you in order to thrive.

Dr. Cowles and other experts offer the following suggestions for expressing a complaint effectively.

- Begin at the first level, with the cashier or the store manager. Or ask who handles problems for the store.
- Use objective statements, instead of accusations or blame. For example, with the cashier, say, "I handed you a $100 bill, and I was given about $30 change on a $43 purchase," not, "I think you ripped me off."
- Be reasonable, accurate, and clear about what you want—your money back or an apology, for instance. Provide the facts and ask for a response.
- Follow with your own nondestructive interpretation, taking responsibility for your own assumptions: "I assume it was because you miscounted," not "I think you pocketed the money." Even if you suspect otherwise, you give the cashier an out.
- Politely say how you feel. "I'm really annoyed that I had to come back here" or "I'm really uncomfortable that I have to bring this up."
- If you don't get a positive response, continue up the company's ladder. Ask to speak to a district manager, or request a corporate telephone number or address and call or write a letter.
- Contact the Federal Consumer Information Center in Pueblo, Colorado, which offers a *Consumer Action Handbook* of more than 650 corporate headquarters— from AAMCO Transmissions to Zenith Packard Bell—and how to reach them. The 148-page handbook can be viewed or ordered free online at www.pueblo.gsa.gov. (Or call the center toll-free at 800-688-9889.) The handbook also gives tips on how to write a letter of complaint.

Road Rage

On her way back to work, Carolyn is cruising along at a comfortable speed when—out of nowhere, it seems—a bright red sport utility vehicle appears in her rearview mirror and bears down on her bumper, headlights snapping on and off.

Getting the Most from Office Meetings

Committee meetings drain you when little is accomplished and you feel you're wasting your time. If you're attending meetings that feel unproductive, speak frankly to your boss and offer to help the group look at the process or find positive solutions.

When all else fails and you're herded into the mandatory "boredom room," look within yourself for some energizing solutions. Imagine feeling energy come up through your spine, walking through a fog into the cool air, shaking the dust off your body, or literally sweeping the cobwebs from your head.

Pick an energy center in your body—your stomach or head—and imagine it's a battery that's being recharged with every breath you take. Breathe deeply and picture yourself elsewhere for a few seconds. Exhale slowly and feel the exhilaration of that mental break. Just don't drift too far, or the meeting might be over when you return!

Experts consulted: Susan Heitler, Ph.D., psychologist and author of *Depression: A Disorder of Power*, Denver, and Angela Stroup, R.N., certified hypnotherapist, mentor/coach, and assistant professor of family and community medicine, Eastern Virginia Medical School, Norfolk

Hey, she's driving at the speed limit in the middle lane. What is she supposed to do? She taps her brakes lightly; she has read that this is an effective way to alert another driver that he is following too closely.

But the driver remains on her tail and then, without any signal, swerves to her right, races past her, and returns to the middle lane, just in front of Carolyn's sedan.

Her heart races. She's furious and half tempted to ride his bumper. Luckily, she doesn't, because within seconds he comes to a complete stop. Carolyn barely has time to brake, nearly plowing into the SUV, which then speeds down the highway and out of sight.

She is wearing her seat belt, so she's physically unhurt, but emotionally consumed. She feels woozy, as though the blood has drained from her head. Her hands and legs quiver like loose shingles in a storm.

Tears spilling down her cheeks, she pulls off on the first exit to calm herself. She has seen aggressive drivers before; she's heard about road rage. But she's never experienced anything like this.

Not responding in anger is wise on Carolyn's part, says Stroup. More than 1,500 people are killed or injured each year as a result of aggressive driving, according to a report from the AAA Foundation for Traffic Safety.

If you find yourself in a situation like Carolyn's, don't let your anger get the best of you. Instead, try some techniques to regain your composure, such as the eye roll. First, with your eyes closed, roll your eyeballs up as if you were attempting to look at your forehead. Breathe in deeply through your nose. Exhale; then lower your eyes (still closed) and feel the wave of relaxation flow through your body.

Practice the eye roll again, only this time think of a word that conjures pleasant images—babies, snow, roses, dew—as you release your breath. See and smell and feel the image the word brings to mind.

Another breathing technique, says Stroup, is to inhale through your nose and then, as you're exhaling, push out all those negative emotions along with your breath with an audible "Ha-a-a-aa."

After such a frightening experience, renew yourself with affirmations, such as "I'm okay," "I'm safe," or "I'm in control." Remember, your mind believes what you tell it. Then, as you pull back onto the highway, envision a divine protector guiding you safely home, or an impervious bubble around your car.

One woman who fears flying told Stroup that she imagines angels holding up the wings of the plane as it takes off, carrying it safely through the air and gently bringing it back to the ground.

Finding Delight in Delays

After an exhausting afternoon, Carolyn decides to skip the grocery store. The next day, Saturday, as she finally makes her way there and searches for a parking spot, she realizes she'll still have time to bake the cookies before Jocelyn's slumber party.

But she's used to shopping on Sunday nights, when the stores are nearly empty. She had forgotten that Saturday mornings are one of the busiest times for supermarkets.

So by the time she scoops up her purchases and hits the express lane, there are at least a dozen people in it. And she is sure that the woman in the front has nearly half a cart full of groceries.

The other lines snake back into the store's aisles, creating a traffic jam and confusion. Just when she thinks things can't get any worse, the cashier starts fumbling with the register tape and calls for assistance.

Carolyn waits, but inside she seethes. "How could this

cashier be so inept?" she fumes. "My day is ruined. I'll never shop here again."

But Carolyn does have other options, says Dr. Quillian. Recognizing that we have choices is important because acting on them won't leave our energy sapped from pent-up fury.

- She could find the manager and calmly ask that another line be opened.
- She could decide the groceries aren't worth the wait and leave, purchasing already baked cookies elsewhere and saving herself the time of making her own.
- She could wait, practice her deep breathing, and enjoy the few minutes she's been given. Yes, *given*, as in gift. Then she could pick up one of those decorating magazines at the checkout to browse through. And instead of bemoaning her bad judgment in picking the wrong line, she should realize that maybe she picked the right line. "Maybe this is the line she's supposed to be in," says Stroup. "Maybe this is time for her to reflect on something pleasant." Like her dinner out tonight.

Six Keys to Better Service

Saturday night finally arrives. Carolyn has been so looking forward to dinner out with Ben, his coworker Joe, and Joe's wife, Shirley.

She's surprised, though, to learn that Joe and Shirley have selected a popular restaurant where reservations aren't accepted and where Saturday waits in summer can stretch to an hour or more.

Additionally, Joe and Shirley have brought their 5-year-old daughter, Destiny, because the couple's babysitter backed out.

Just as she suspected, the restaurant line snakes out the door. Although they're told the wait will be only 40 minutes, it's 2 hours before they're seated. By now, Destiny is beyond hunger. She's tired and whiny. Carolyn can relate. She aches to snap at the waitress even as the server appears at the table within seconds, a huge bowl of hush puppies in hand and ready to take drink and appetizer orders.

Carolyn is pleasantly surprised at the prompt service, but she's still not completely convinced that choosing this restaurant wasn't a mistake.

By the time the waitress returns to take their order, Destiny and her adult companions are happily munching on hush puppies.

Then Shirley asks if Destiny's dinner could be delivered first. She requests that her own meal be prepared without salt and minus the scallops and scallop juice to which she is allergic. Ben asks that his "fried fish platter" be broiled and another vegetable substituted for the potato.

Carolyn is amazed when the server replies, "Absolutely!"

She's so used to getting bad service from "incompetent" wait staff and leaving restaurants tired or angry that she has never thought to spell out her own needs so clearly.

"A lot of people don't even think to ask," says Gail Glass, a waitress for 13 years at Lynnhaven Fish House in Virginia Beach. But in many full-service restaurants, she says, the waitress is your ally, especially if you have special requests.

Glass has learned to tune in to her customers. She almost instinctively knows when they're feeling grouchy from a wait or downright famished. In her early waitressing days, however, those encounters were so exhausting for her that she sometimes went home teary-eyed.

"You can get customers out of their bad moods if you're receptive," she says of skilled servers. Now she can almost see when a group is reenergized, and that's invigorating for her, too.

Glass offers several suggestions for avoiding energy-draining frustration when dining out.

- Know what you want in terms of service before choosing a restaurant. If you don't want to wait 2 hours on a Saturday night, pick an eatery that takes reservations.
- Always tell the waitress how she can best serve you. Are there foods you can't eat? A particular order in which you'd like the food to be served? Do you have only an hour before the movie starts? She's not a mind reader.
- If a meal arrives tepid or prepared incorrectly, say so. A good restaurant will replace it pronto and offer a bowl of soup or appetizer while you wait.
- If the service or food is unacceptable and the waitress doesn't comply, ask to see a manager. But express your needs clearly, Dr. Quillian says. What do you want? Your money back? A voucher for another meal? But be fair; don't eat half the cold fries and then demand a refund.
- Fill out the comment card, which is usually on the table or at the front of the restaurant, to indicate whether the experience was poor or superb.
- Relax. After all, isn't that the point of a restaurant meal? "It really is okay to wait 5 minutes," says Dr. Cowles. "It's okay for the server to make a mistake; it's okay for that tolerance zone of waiting time to be relaxed once in a while."

The New Workplace

It's the school nurse calling: "Jocelyn is ill. Can you pick her up?"

Carolyn freezes on the other end of her phone. She glances at the pile of work teetering on her desk. "Not today," she moans inside. But ever the competent mother, she calmly says, "I'll be right there."

She nearly tiptoes into her boss's office, praying he'll be in a good mood. And although she gets the go-ahead to leave, it's accompanied by that suspicious, one-raised-eyebrow look she hates. She ignores it. She has no other choice; Ben's away on business again.

On the way home from the middle school, with Jocelyn moaning in the backseat from painful menstrual cramps, Carolyn's beeper chirps. It's her boss, of course, and the terse message on the display tells her to check her e-mail from home and hurry back to the office—he needs the monthly budget compilations immediately. Once home, Carolyn quickly checks her e-mail and gives Jocelyn an ibuprofen fix. Then she's back on the road. She grips the steering wheel with white-knuckled hands as she drives—

Asleep on the Job

Sleep specialists say workplace snoozes can energize you, increase your performance, and decrease the number of mistakes you make. As little as 5 to 10 minutes of shut-eye can provide the jolt you need, says Camille Anthony, coauthor of *The Art of Napping at Work*.

Some companies set aside special rooms for napping. A few companies even offer office or cubicle tents designed for employees to curl up in when a drowsy period hits. "Whether employers realize it or not, there is napping going on in work areas," says Anthony. Employees who don't have the luxury of a private room complete with a couch and a cozy blanket find a way—they take a quick nap on, under, or beside their desks, in the bathroom, or in their cars.

"Not everyone wants a nap room or will use it every day, but it should be available," says Anthony. "You just can't be creative when you're tired."

partially because she's in a hurry but also because of the mounting pressures of work and home pushing down on her shoulders.

It's a common scenario for millions of working mothers—a never-ending workplace where the traditional boundaries between home and job have blurred to the point of indistinctness. Forget 8-hour days; these days we're working 24/7.

To escape burnout and maintain excellence on all fronts, you have to take care of yourself, says Filomena Warihay, Ph.D., president of Take Charge Consultants, an international management training and organizational development firm in Downingtown, Pennsylvania. "The key to success in this rapidly changing business world is knowing what to stop—as well as what to start."

The Demands of a Changing Workplace

In 1960, a panel of government authorities predicted big changes in the workplace because of budding technological advances. Number one: more free time. Boy, were they ever wrong. Granted, technology has simplified some aspects of our lives, but it's not shaving any hours off our workdays. In fact, we're working 3 hours longer each week than in 1980, we're taking 20 percent less vacation time, and the phrase "leisure time" has been tossed in the backs of our closets like the suits bearing the same name. "Expectations have changed along with the tools and technology," says Kathleen Conroy, vice president of client relations at employeesavings.com, a work/life solution provider in Seattle. "We're expected to be on call virtually around the clock."

Organizational changes have occurred along with technological advances. Companies are downsizing, temporary employees are replacing full-time ones, and we get raises based on our contributions to company profits rather than our tenure. "The old psychological contract between employer and worker, where the worker gives her loyalty and the employer guarantees long-term employment, is dead," says Dr. Warihay. Today the employee brings a skill, and the employer provides employment as long as that skill is needed.

"Changes in the workplace are both positive and negative," says Sharon Keys Seal, certified professional business coach and president of Coaching Concepts in Baltimore. "They're positive in that many companies are looking at the 'whole employee' and trying to accommodate needs like security, safety, and flextime. They're negative in that employees are expected to work longer and harder."

Workplace changes have been particularly hard on working women, who now make up about 60 percent of the workforce. Although some women's magazines glorify the woman who made her first million before age 30, jogs and swims daily, has three kids, and works more than 60 hours a week, the reality is that she provides an unrealistic ideal for the rest of us, contributing to our own burnout.

In addition, our values are changing. We're rewarded much less for an afternoon at the zoo with the kids than for a productive day at the office, so it's no surprise many of us choose to devote our time to the latter. The result: less time spent with our families and friends. In fact, our lifestyles discourage our making a priority of things like our families, friends, health, volunteer work, and vacations—areas of life that are crucial for personal and societal well-being, says Barbara J. Distler, Psy.D., a licensed clinical psychologist in Chicago.

These changes are only a part of the mix that is pushing more and more working women to burnout. Other factors include the following:

The perfection factor. A survey from Northwestern National Life Insurance Company showed that female employees suffer more from burnout and stress-related illnesses than men, and they're more likely to quit their jobs. "Part of the reason is that many women grew up in an era when they had to be better than men in the same position to survive," says Dr. Warihay. "So they confuse perfection with performance."

The dual-role factor. Although the number of working women is at an all-time high, no equivalent household revolution has emerged to counteract this increase. Nearly one-third of us earn more than our partners, yet we still do the bulk of housework and child rearing. Then, too, more working women than ever are single or are taking care of elderly parents. "Many women feel conflicted—there are greater opportunities in the work world, yet there are more personal demands on them," says Dr. Warihay. Luckily, adds Conroy, a new generation of young men is sharing more of the housework, but we probably won't see the results of this trend for a while.

The blurry-line factor. When you got the laptop on the first day of your new job, you probably thought, "What a perk!" But with that perk came a hidden message: "Use me at home." The Internet expands the average woman's workdays further—we can connect at all hours with e-mail, electronic files, and coworkers around the world. "Because it has become so much harder to protect our time away from work, we are at a much greater risk of burning out," says Dr. Distler.

The I-hate-my-job factor. The amount of joy we get from our jobs has a bearing on whether or not we burn out, says Dr. Warihay. Numerous things help our workplace happiness. Good relationships with subordinates, colleagues, and superiors are important. A feeling of control over your job, where you have a clear picture of what is expected of you, how to do it, and where it fits into the company as a whole, is also important. Stimulating work is an obvious, yet necessary, plus.

On the flip side, things that jeopardize job satisfaction include a difficult boss who behaves unpredictably, places you in frustrating situations, and damages your self-confidence. Shaky job security—not knowing whether your job will be there tomorrow after a possible merger or acquisition—has a similar effect.

The I-have-a-life factor. Women who don't have children are experiencing work burnout, too, in part because they are sometimes expected to pick up the slack of the

Are You a Workaholic?

Feel like you may be just a bit too caught up in your work? Give yourself this test.

Check off all of the following statements that fairly regularly apply to you. If you check at least two items, you may be on the way to wearing a workaholic badge. If four or more items apply to you, you're already there. Read over the tips in this chapter on how to tackle work burnout.

I take work home with me.

I put family obligations after work responsibilities.

I feel like the company will go under without me.

I think I can handle any workload, no matter how large.

I would rather do the work myself than delegate it.

I feel I can do my job better than others in my department.

I check my e-mail at least every hour when I am at work, even if I'm not expecting an important message.

I work more than 40 hours in a week.

I call the office when I'm on vacation.

I think about work when I'm at home.

Expert consulted: Sharon Keys Seal, a certified professional business coach and president of Coaching Concepts in Baltimore

working mothers, says Carlla Smith, Ph.D., professor of industrial and organizational psychology at Bowling Green State University in Ohio. For example, the working woman without children may be asked to change meeting times to accommodate the working mother. Hence, she has less time to spend with her friends or family.

Danger Signs of Burnout

"It's essential to recognize the difference between a slump and burnout," says Dr. Warihay. True burnout is a form of depression, the kind of stress that isn't fixed by a relaxing weekend on the beach.

Burnout also has implications beyond our own lives. "The more we suffer from burnout, the more health and emotional difficulties we'll be faced with as a society," says Dr. Distler.

Here are some of the signs of burnout.

Behavioral red flags. Changes in behavior are the earliest signs of occupational stress. In the first stages of burnout, you may begin to avoid coworkers, ignore work responsibilities, pay less attention to your appearance, and make mistakes more frequently. "You may also find yourself becoming irritable, defensive, arrogant, and insubordinate," notes Dr. Warihay. Eventually, dramatic behavioral changes may occur. "You may be a neat person and then suddenly become really sloppy, for example," she says. Or you may find yourself indulging in a nightly cocktail and cigarette after years of not drinking or smoking.

Emotional warning signs. If you can't remember the last moment you had to yourself, you may be on the cusp of burnout. Feelings of being overworked, unappreciated, and out of control at work are additional signals. Difficulties with your spouse or children are another sign. "When you're burned-out, you're likely to become anxious, insecure, sad, and preoccupied, and you may no longer get pleasure out of activities you once enjoyed," says Dr. Warihay.

Physical symptoms. Emotional stress affects us physically. For example, stress is a bigger culprit in elevated cholesterol levels than is a diet high in cheese and eggs. In fact, some tax accountants' cholesterol levels rise sharply just before April 15, then fall back to normal shortly after the tax filing deadline. In addition, if you're burned-out, you're more likely to experience fatigue, sleep disturbances, appetite changes, indigestion, headaches, frequent illnesses, and sexual dysfunction, says Dr. Warihay.

Eight Ways to End Burnout

The remedy for burnout is not as obvious as the problem itself. "Some women decide to quit altogether and stay home," says Dr. Smith. But many of us can't afford that option. And there's always the fear that if we drop out of the workforce, our only option for reentry will be in a lower position.

If you're feeling burned-out and quitting isn't an option, you need to look for other options. "If you wait till the point of illness or depression, you'll limit your alternatives," says Dr. Smith. Here are a few suggestions.

Declutter your workload. Take an objective look at your tasks, and clean out the unnecessary. "Every month, try to stop doing at least two things—no one is likely to even notice," says Dr. Warihay. For example, erase all forwarded e-mail jokes and chain letters before opening them, or transcribe only those portions of the budget meeting that really matter. And finish your projects both at work and at home.

List your to-dos. "We feel more energized when we actually get things done," notes Conroy. Start your workday by writing down your tasks and how long you have to do them. For example, "I have to make five phone calls and type three reports between 2:00 and 5:00." Then, each time you cross something off, reward yourself with an energizing activity. When you finish a report, call your spouse to give your brain a change of pace, or grab a quick snack with a coworker.

Exercise for work. "If you ride a bike 5 miles on Sunday, filing on Monday will seem like a piece of cake," says Janet O'Mahony, M.D., a physician in internal medicine at Mercy Medical Center in Baltimore. "But if your most strenuous daily activity is walking to the vending machine, you'll feel exhausted just answering the phones." Exercisers miss fewer days of work, are more often in a good mood, and are mentally and physically healthier overall than their sedentary coworkers.

Eat for energy. For maximum energy at work, eat something in the morning (even if it's only a piece of fruit or a granola bar). For lunch, a meal brought from home, such as a tuna fish sandwich or stir-fry leftovers from last night's dinner, is usually more nutritious than fast food eaten on the go. And since most of us don't eat dinner until after 6, a version of afternoon tea is a good idea. "Bring in some fruit or yogurt to eat in the afternoon," Dr. O'Mahony suggests.

Laugh it off. "Bad days aren't so bad if you can laugh at adversity," says Dr. O'Mahony. This doesn't mean you shouldn't take your job seriously, but women who can see the hidden humor in a printer paper jam or an unreasonably grouchy coworker tend to view potentially stressful situations more objectively.

Make friends at the coffee machine. Social support is a major stress reducer at work, and studies show that women with work comrades are absent less often. "Make it a point to rub shoulders with the people at work who energize you," recommends Conroy. Grab lunch with them, or spend a few minutes at the end of the day catching up with each other.

Synthesize your life. "Efficiency means getting more done by doing less work," says Dr. O'Mahony. Have a routine you follow every day. For example, pack lunches and iron clothes the night before, and use that time in the morning to relax and energize yourself with a cup of herbal tea and an engrossing magazine before you leave for work. At work, keep things neat and orderly. Maintain an alphabetized filing cabinet, put your scattered desk papers into piles so your disorganization doesn't stare you in the face, and periodically dust off your work space so you work on a clean slate. "When you're organized, you don't have to waste time looking

Desk-Job Fatigue

Funny how tired you can get sitting at a desk all day. But staying put for 8 hours *is* fatiguing. And if your daily tasks are somewhat mundane, you may not have enough mental action to keep you energized. Further, computer-induced eyestrain can worsen the problem.

To keep from dragging yourself home at the end of the day, move around whenever you can. Get away from your desk at lunch and walk around the building. You don't have to walk for an hour—just 10 minutes here and there when you get a chance will help.

If it's not convenient to leave your work area, swivel your chair away from your computer and do some stretches and deep breathing. If you have an office mate or two, have one of you lead stretching exercises every hour or so—it will build camaraderie as it energizes you. If your office approves, listen to some uplifting music on headphones while you type.

Expert consulted: Cheryl Dellasega, Ph.D., associate director of research in general internal medicine, Pennsylvania State University's Hershey Medical Center

for things, and you generally do a better job," says Dr. O'Mahony.

Leave without a trace. Periodic rest and relaxation is very important for a healthy body and work attitude. If you can't afford a vacation to Fiji, try a camping trip or head to the beach—someplace where you're not wired to your cell phone or the Internet. Although it's often hard to fit vacations into our busy schedules, "you need to draw the line in the sand at some point, just say no, and go," Conroy says.

The Energizing Work Environment

Studies show that we're in our cubicles for one-third of our waking hours. So make the atmosphere there as pleasant as possible. Here are some suggestions for sprucing up your cube.

Make it cozy. Put some throw pillows on your chairs. Bring in a small desktop fountain—the gurgling will soothe you as you work. Plants also make a nice addition, and they give off energizing oxygen. "Fresh cut flowers are visually pleasing, and they smell good," says Conroy. So splurge on a bunch or ask for a weekly flower delivery as a birthday present.

Invigorate with color. Warm colors, like reds, oranges, and yellows, provide energy. Red makes our hearts beat faster, and yellow is thought to make us more creative and communicative. In addition, green helps us concentrate. On the other hand, whites, blues, and blacks can have a depressing effect. You probably don't have the freedom to repaint your work space, but you can probably hang an energizing red and yellow poster or painting.

Put motivation in view. Decorate your work space with items that stimulate and energize you, such as paintings, inspirational sayings, and pictures of your family trip to Disney World. Collect meaningful quotes and feature a new one each morning on your bulletin board. "Even using an interesting handmade pottery coffee mug versus the company-issued Styrofoam cups can make a big difference," notes Seal.

Should You Quit?

The decision to stay in a job or go elsewhere depends on the situation at hand, says Kathleen Conroy, vice president of client relations at employeesavings.com, a work/life solution provider in Seattle. Some scenarios do necessitate an immediate change. But if you're considering a switch because your company is going through a rough period or you're bored, think twice.

Frequent job changers are usually viewed favorably in smaller start-up and technology companies, but larger, more mature organizations look at them with suspicion. "The ability to see through challenging situations, overcome obstacles, and creatively problem-solve are all demonstrated by a long-term career track within a given company, particularly if you're progressing and being promoted," says Conroy.

Instead of immediately reaching for the want ads, conduct some self-analysis. Consider whether it's your job that's making you unhappy, or the way you're perceiving it. "Make sure you've done everything you can to improve the surroundings you're presently in, because the grass usually isn't greener on the other side," says Conroy. You may leave because of low pay in your present job only to find that a slightly higher salary somewhere else means a whole lot more hours.

Energize with effervescence. Pleasant fragrances stimulate nerves in our bodies that promote wakefulness. Peppermint and citrus, for example, specifically have been shown to increase energy and concentration. So put a little bowl of dried peppermint or lemon rind on your desk, or use some citrus or peppermint essential oil. The diffusers that plug into electrical outlets also provide a nice scent.

Create ideal illumination. If possible, light should be on your desk and your task; lights from above or behind force you to work in a shadow. Find out whether you may have the overhead lights turned off and bring in a desk lamp from home. Lightbulbs that are red-yellow are best at boosting mood.

Mold your mood with music. Listening to music while you work can both relax and energize you, says Cheryl Dellasega, Ph.D., associate director of research in general internal medicine at Pennsylvania State University's Hershey Medical Center. If you need a boost, plug in some energizing tunes; if you're feeling frazzled, soothing music can calm your nerves. Just be courteous of your neighbors, and wear headphones if necessary.

How Companies Cope with Burnout

The litany of work woes mentioned so far may sound overwhelming. But try not to get too discouraged—changes are in the works. "Employers are becoming more understanding because they themselves are experiencing the strain of balancing work and home," says Dr. Smith. Some employers offer support services such as life-improvement seminars, on-site child care, and flextime, and they welcome their employees to come to them with problems. "Although a workplace reorganization may not be happening fast enough for someone in the middle of all this, things certainly are changing," Dr. Smith says.

In the meantime, take advantage of what is available to you. For example, if you're having trouble with a supervisor or coworker, talk to someone in human resources or ask your boss how you can do a better job, says Dr. O'Mahony. The other thing to keep in mind is that your job is *just* your job. "There are clearly other things that are more important in life," she points out. "If your job were great all the time, you wouldn't be paid to go there."

On the Home Front

Carolyn glances at her watch, realizing with a start that it's already 5:30. She needs to leave work immediately to get Michael to soccer practice.

As soon as she puts her key in the door at home, however, her stomach begins churning. The blast of rap music that meets her in the living room, coupled with the sight of unwashed breakfast dishes in the sink, is enough to start her head pounding. She yells up the stairs for Michael to turn down the music and get ready for soccer. Then she throws the mail on the ever-growing stack on the hall table and heads for the kitchen, picturing the inside of her freezer and wondering if there is anything in it for dinner. She sets aside a package of frozen hamburger and yells again for Michael to hurry up.

Thus begins her evening.

During the next 4 hours, Carolyn drives to and from the soccer field twice, fixes dinner for the family, cleans up the kitchen, does two loads of laundry, calls her mother to say hello, searches frantically for the permission slip Michael needs for school, and checks Jocelyn's homework, resulting in a tense discussion about why leaving reports until the last minute is a generally bad idea.

By 9 P.M., Carolyn is exhausted but still working; she irons Ben's shirts while watching her favorite TV program. She keeps thinking that she should straighten the house or at least tackle that pile of mail and newspapers, but she just doesn't have the energy.

It should come as no surprise that life on the home front can be even more draining than life in the workplace. If we're lucky, we feel some degree of control at work. The schedule is predictable, our duties and responsibilities are spelled out, the chain of command clear. And at least we know *someone* is going to empty the trash and vacuum the floor.

At home, it's a different story. The schedule changes daily, no one wants responsibility, and on some days it seems no one—or everyone—is in charge. Plus, our to-do lists are endless and repetitive. After all, you never finish washing dishes or doing laundry, the way you finish a report. So, for many of us, home life spins out of control, draining us of energy.

Our home life has contracted, says author Cheryl Mendelson in *Home Comforts: The Art and Science of Keeping House.* As we clean less, cook less, and entertain at home less, we risk losing the knack. Increasingly, we become strangers in our own homes and lose that sense of solace that a home provides.

But you can bring your home life out of chaos and clutter. Below are ways to establish a peaceful home where you and your family can regroup, relax, and refresh.

Exorcise the Expectation Demon

There are actually researchers out there who get paid to study housework. Thanks to them, we have research to back up what we've known since we got married: We do more around the house than he does. About 60 percent more, according to one Ohio State University study. In fact, women list housework as one of the leading causes of fatigue. Overall, we're doing two-thirds of the household work, ranging from cleaning the house to scheduling the kids' dentist appointments.

Why, then, do our standards still include such things as a sparkling refrigerator and weekly dusting? Who actually sees the inside of our refrigerators? Are we bad mothers if there are fuzzy things in the back and spilled juice on the shelves? Of course not.

"You have to get rid of the idea of perfect and best and adopt the idea of 'this works,'" says Margaret Sanik, Ph.D.,

Technology: Energizer or Energy Zapper?

While technology has simplified some tasks for us, it has also blurred the boundaries between home and office and made our home lives a maze of multitasking, says Helen Seltzer, president and chief operating officer of MessageClick, a high-tech unified messaging service.

Used with restraint, however, technology can be a godsend to the energy- and time-starved woman. There are three keys to successfully integrating technology into your life, Seltzer says: It must be simple, provide information on demand, and be mobile. Mobility is important particularly to working mothers.

Here are a few ways today's wired world can make your life easier.

• Bank online, including having your paycheck directly deposited and bills automatically paid.

a time allocation expert and associate professor of consumer sciences at Ohio State University in Columbus. "The first thing you have to realize is that the world doesn't fall apart if all those expectations are not met."

Instead, you should focus on what really matters to your family. When Dr. Sanik first married, for instance, she folded her husband's socks and underwear. "Why'd you do that?" he asked her. Now she learns what's really important to him and concentrates on the things that are appreciated, such as home-cooked meals.

If your children would be just as happy with slice-and-bake chocolate chip cookies, don't knock yourself out making the from-scratch ones. If you're the only one who ever sees the upstairs bathroom, leave the cleaning for

- Shop online, having gifts wrapped and mailed directly to the recipient.
- Stay connected with e-mail. It has largely replaced letter writing and phoning, because it's quicker and not as intrusive, Seltzer says.
- Cut down on clutter. Spend a weekend entering into your computer addresses, telephone numbers, birthdays, anniversaries, and other annual events, in addition to time-saving lists such as instructions for house sitters and what to pack for holidays. Draw up a sample grocery list you can print out each week and keep on the refrigerator, circling each item that's needed.
- Keep in touch via cell phones, pagers, laptops, personal organizing devices (such as Palm Pilots), online fax services, and unified messaging services.

next week. Dr. Sanik doesn't check her children's home-work, and she still has two straight-A students. But, she cautions, one size doesn't fit all; know what works for your family.

Other expectations to jettison:

- Polishing silver. Keep it under wraps so it doesn't tarnish.
- Drying dishes. That's what air is for.
- Balanced meals. Every meal doesn't have to have a vegetable and a starch. It doesn't matter when you get your five veggies a day, just as long as you get them.
- Fund-raising. Forget selling candy and gift wrap for the PTA. Write a check instead.
- Ironing. You have four choices: Don't buy clothes that need ironing; get everything dry-cleaned; pull clothes out of the dryer when they're still slightly damp; accept the wrinkled look.
- And the golden rule of lowered expectations: If it isn't dirty or can't be seen, don't clean it.

Make Housework a Family Affair

Unfortunately, there's only so far you can go with your new, lowered expectations before a dirty, messy house becomes more of an energy drainer than cleaning it would be.

You have two choices: Hire a housekeeper or enlist the family. If you choose the first, you can skip down to the next section in this chapter. Otherwise, here's how to delegate.

"Mothers who feel like they have to do everything for their kids are really burdening themselves," says Catherine A. Chambliss, Ph.D., psychology professor and department chair at Ursinus College in Collegeville, Pennsylvania. And they're not doing their kids any favors. By the time children are teenagers, they should know how to cook, clean, do laundry, and in general have responsibility for most aspects of their lives, she says. "We should view the development of independence as one of the prime goals of mothering," Dr. Chambliss says.

And don't go lighter on the boys. A Swarthmore College study shows that the chore gender gap—the difference between the time girls and boys spend on housework—doubles from 2 hours to 4 between the freshman and senior years in high school. That leaves more time for the boys to spend on extracurricular and leisure activities.

To get the kids and your husband to do their fair share, you have to get their attention first. You can try the civilized way: setting up a meeting and calmly explaining the facts of 32 loads of laundry a week, two bathrooms to clean, and a dog that hasn't been bathed since your high schooler was in diapers. Request a second meeting if necessary. If, by the third meeting, your family still doesn't catch on, a more dramatic approach may be required: You could go on strike or picket the house. Somehow, says Susan Schenkel, Ph.D., a clinical psychologist in Cambridge, Massachusetts, you need to let them know the ways they're making it needlessly hard for you and how they can help you. "Change can take time, but it pays to be persistent."

Now that you have their attention, where do you start?

Assign chores. When it comes to household chores, the more consistent you are as a parent, the quicker your kids will comply, says Deniece Schofield, a home-management consultant and author of *Confessions of a Happily Organized Family.* Routine household chores teach a child about responsibility, about family, about participation in groups, and many other valuable life skills.

Even a 2-year-old can pick up her toys. Starting with

young children, have them spend 5 minutes a day straightening their rooms. You may have to physically be in the room with them at first, but you can sit on the bed and read a magazine or return a phone call while they do the work. If you start your 3-year-old sorting laundry, by the time he's 11 or 12, he should be measuring out the fabric softener and spraying on stain remover.

By the time your children are 8 or 9, they can vacuum, dust, set and clear the table, help with preparing a meal, unload the dishwasher or wash the dishes, and clean a bathroom. Once they hit their teens, they can do almost any housework you can.

Schedule it. Recognize that housework is an infinite task. If you don't make a schedule and stick to it, you'll never get free. For example, do laundry only 1 or 2 days a week. To eliminate constant interruptions from someone looking for clean socks, let everyone in the family know the schedule, recommends Schofield.

Appoint an assistant. In large families, name young assistants for a week to help with such chores as laundry, kitchen duties, and yard work. This person can also be the designated gofer. Rotate the duties and post a schedule.

Create a card file. To enlist her children, organizing guru Barbara Hemphill of Raleigh, North Carolina, wrote each household chore on an index card and assigned it points based on difficulty and desirability. For example, vacuuming the family room might be 5 points and cleaning the bathrooms 15 points. Each child had an envelope with his or her name on it and points assigned based on age and ability. The children chose which tasks they wanted to do each week to reach their assigned points and put those cards in their envelopes. If the tasks weren't completed by noon Saturday, the child lost TV privileges for a week. "It gave the kids control over what they did and when they did it—and the kids monitored

Sex: The Super Energizer

For many, sex is just one more thing to squeeze into a busy day. But it's worth the effort, says Linda De Villers, Ph.D., a certified sex therapist and psychologist based in El Segundo, California. "Sex can help you maintain a sense of sanity and balance in your hectic life."

Making sex a priority vitalizes the marriage as well as the body. And orgasms release tension, Dr. De Villers says. Our bodies produce endorphins, the "feel-good" hormones that are the body's natural painkiller, leaving us a little euphoric.

Our bodies also release oxytocin during orgasm. This hormone may be involved in adult bonding. A preliminary study at the University of California, San Francisco, suggests oxytocin is associated with maintaining healthy relationships and healthy psychological boundaries, both of which could have energizing effects. Social situations may also induce oxytocin release, and the presence of the hormone may make good relationships more rewarding.

And let's not forget that sex is exercise—good for the heart and the muscles. On an emotional level, sex improves our self-esteem and increases our intimacy and communication with our partners, says Barbara Bartlik, M.D., clinical assistant professor of psychiatry at Weill Medical College of Cornell University in New York City.

The question is when to find the time. Dr. De Villers recommends setting aside time to make it a nourishing experience. A warm shower or bath can help a busy woman make the transition, and a nap can be the perfect finish.

each other," says Hemphill, author of the *Taming the Paper Tiger* books.

Create a chore chart. This can be as simple as a handwritten, color-coded chart that divides chores among family members and lists daily, weekly, and monthly responsibilities, or it can be a fancy spreadsheet. Rotate chores weekly or monthly so no one tires of them. Check out the Internet site www.shiftschedules.com to download a free weekly family chore spreadsheet.

Be absolutely, unequivocally clear. This is obviously necessary with young children, but no less so with teenagers. Tell a 13-year-old to wash the dishes and he'll likely wash only those dishes in the sink, not the ones on the counter or table. Nor will he wipe the counters or clean out the sink. Write it out, if necessary, but don't leave it open to interpretation.

Make it a family affair. Some chores are more tolerable if tackled together. Host a clothes-folding session, where everyone folds clothes while watching a favorite video or TV show. Designate a time of the day or week, like 5 minutes before dinner, when everyone puts away anything left out of place that day. Or establish a Sunday-night pickup party, when everyone goes around the house putting away the weekend detritus and finishes up with a bowl of ice cream. You can use TV commercials for a little cleaning or straightening competition—who can pick up all their things first, clean a mirror quickest, or empty all the trash cans on one floor before the program resumes?

Create a ransom box. Kids won't clean up? At the end of the day (or week) collect every wayward object in sight and stash it in a box or bag. On Saturday the owners may regain possession by doing a chore or paying a ransom for each item they reclaim.

On the husband front:

Put it in writing. The more you nag him, the less likely it is that he'll do what you want. So make a list on Friday night of every chore you both need to accomplish on the weekend, sign the ones you can handle, and get him to sign off on the ones he can do. He may not take on as much as you'd hoped, but at least he has signed on to the team. A bonus: You'll get better response from the kids if you present a united front.

Play to their strengths. If your he-man is a klutz when it comes to hammer and nails but earns a good living, is willing to run errands, and chauffeurs the kids, count your blessings and stop feeling like a martyr for doing things you're good at. You may be surprised at how much more cooperation you get once you quit nagging.

Housework Hints

Now that you have your workforce organized, there are ways to get the job done faster and better, leaving you with more energy for the other things on your to-do list.

Assemble supplies. Keep a tote of cleaning supplies in a central location on each floor of your home, near where they'll be needed. For instance, every bathroom cabinet should be stocked with bathroom cleaner, glass cleaner, paper towels, and a sponge, and the hall closet should have dusting spray and rags. You can pick up a cheap vacuum cleaner at a garage sale for the upstairs.

Stop dirt at the door. Encourage family and friends to leave their shoes at the door; have a handy basket nearby. To trap dirt, put a mat on each side of doors leading to the outside.

Simplify bedding. Using a comforter instead of a bedspread saves valuable seconds on bed making each morning. After you wash sheets, fold a matched set and store it inside a matching pillowcase. That way, there's only one thing to grab when it's time to change the sheets.

Separate laundry once. Once a week, put three laundry baskets in the hall and have all family members sort their laundry into colors, whites, and delicates. When the laundry is clean, pile each person's stuff into an individual basket and leave it in that person's room.

Line wastebaskets with grocery bags. If you're using plastic bags, for quick changes keep a few extras stuffed in the bottom of each wastebasket.

Make a sock drawer. Designate one drawer for all the white socks in the house. Then just throw them in, unmatched, and let people pull them out as needed.

Clutter Control

Clutter is a sign of postponed decisions, says Schofield. In some homes, it's a flashing neon sign, constantly reminding us that our lives are out of control. But you don't need to be a neat freak to want some element of order in your home. The more organized you become, the more time you'll free up for spontaneity and stress-reducing fun. Here's how to invest a little time now so you're free later.

Streamline your stuff. Even the most organized among us always seems to be a bit of a pack rat at heart. We hang on to things we think might be useful *someday*, such as clothing we might wear when we lose 20 pounds. In the meantime, these things get in the way of real life and suck up precious time. Organizing guru Hemphill has a simple solution: "Have nothing in your home that you do not know to be useful, think to be beautiful, or love."

If you want to declutter your house, here's Hemphill's advice. Start with one room, three boxes, and a trash can. In one box put things you must keep; in the second put things you want to give away, sell, or donate; and in the third put things you aren't sure about. Move quickly. When box three is full, seal it and store it. After a year, if you haven't needed anything in it, get rid of it (but don't open it or you risk becoming reattached).

Here are some questions to ask yourself as you sort.

- Is it a duplicate? After all, how many whisks, spatulas, coffee makers, and plastic containers do you really need? For example, must you have bags full of other bags?
- Can you easily find the item or information somewhere else if you get rid of it?
- Are you keeping this because you think it will become valuable? If so, find a collector now, and get rid of it. It probably won't be very valuable in your lifetime anyway.
- Is this a family heirloom? If so, see if there's a family member you can pass it along to. If you plan to will it to someone, why not just give it to that person now to avoid battles after you're gone?
- Is this souvenir really worth saving? Sometimes a picture and a few words in an album will suffice.
- Are you keeping this because you don't want to offend the giver? If the person must know, be honest and admit that it doesn't fit your lifestyle and you passed it along to someone who could really use it.
- What's the worst possible thing that could happen if you don't save this item? This works with everything from clothes and kitchenware to books and papers.

Look forward, not backward. "Today's mail is tomorrow's pile," Hemphill says. If you start by trying to deal with the backlog, you'll never catch up. Move the backlog out of the way and set up a system to start where you are today.

Now you're ready to move on to maintenance.

Toss as you go. Keep a box in every closet of every room. When something doesn't fit or breaks, or you think you could live without it, drop it in. When the box is full, decide what you'll donate and what you'll throw away.

Fill a treasure chest. Put in each closet another box, marked "treasures," to hold all those keepsakes that can quickly take over a dresser or desk.

Recycle. We're talking about those piles of magazines you just can't bear to throw away because they seem so much more substantial than newspapers. Donate them to a hospital, nursing home, or day care center, or just haul them into work and put them in the coffee room for the taking.

Free your refrigerator. Get three-ring binders and some plastic sheet protectors. Put each child's name on a binder, then let the child fill it with special artwork and stories, class pictures, awards, report cards, and other memorabilia that typically clutters up your refrigerator, bulletin board, and walls. For bulky art projects, take a Polaroid picture and include it in the book.

Set up a center. Put all your important papers in one place. It could be a desk in the kitchen or the study, but keep it convenient to the kitchen/family room. Gather a file cabinet and folders, telephone, office supplies, calendar (paper or electronic), clock, stamps, wastebasket, and recycling box. Set up three trays for sorting: "in box," "out box," and "to-file box."

Get the picture. Photographs can quickly morph into a pack rat's worst enemy. If you can't manage to sort them into scrapbooks, just scrawl a few notes on each envelope of pictures when you pick them up. Then put them in lidless shoe boxes. At the end of the year, put into the boxes the appropriate pages from a calendar, providing notes for reference.

File it where you need it. Get a portable plastic file box for the kitchen. It holds about 15 hanging files and can organize things like takeout menus, tickets and invitations to upcoming events, coupons, papers you need to sign, and correspondence to answer. Used in conjunction with a calendar, a hanging file box can clear a lot of clutter and save time.

Keep a calendar. The refrigerator remains the central posting place for many families. Place there a family calendar, an erasable memo board, and a magnetic refrigerator caddy for papers that need signing or immediate attention. If the kids have something that requires parental involvement—such as sports practice or baking for school—make a rule that if it's not on the calendar, you're not obligated to drop everything and take care of it. Calendar codes, such as P for Pending, can remind you to check the hanging file box for more information.

Create and use a personal planner. Start with a bought planner, or custom-design your own using a small looseleaf notebook. Include yearly and daily calendar pages, birthdays and other significant dates, important phone numbers, family clothing sizes, project ideas and notes, and a pouch for short-term papers, such as directions, coupons, and tickets. The notebook will evolve over time depending on your own personal needs, but don't hesitate to add things such as wallpaper, fabric, and paint samples; committee notes and phone lists; reading lists; and memorable thoughts and quotes.

Carry a waiting bag. Fill a bag with things you never seem to have time for, and carry it with you so you can tackle them while stuck in traffic, watching soccer practice, or waiting in a doctor's office. You can include such things as bills to pay, bank statements to balance, reading material, invitations and announcements, thank-you notes, stationery, greeting cards, and craft projects.

Color Your World

Certain colors are associated with certain moods, and a fresh coat of paint can work wonders. Is the kitchen always the most chaotic room of the house? Try blue for a more tranquil, leisurely atmosphere. Family room dark and sunless? Make the most of existing light and warm the atmosphere with white, off-white, or yellow. Cozy up a large, cold room with rich, warm colors like burgundy.

Here's what you can expect from different colors.

- Pink: Soothes and promotes affability and affection
- Yellow: Cheers and energizes
- White: Energizes, unifies, and enlivens other colors
- Black: Strengthens and encourages discipline
- Orange: Cheers; stimulates appetite and conversation
- Red: Stimulates and dramatizes
- Green: Balances, refreshes, encourages emotional growth
- Purple: Comforts, spiritualizes, encourages intuition
- Blue: Relaxes, refreshes, promotes peaceful moods

Conquering Kid Chaos

A 1997 study by researchers at the University of Michigan's Institute for Social Research shows that many children today have 75 percent of their weekdays programmed, an increase from 40 percent in 1981. More than half the time of the children in the study was spent playing organized sports.

This dramatic change in family life is largely related to mothers working outside the home, says Sandra Hofferth, coauthor of a study on how children spend their time.

And while she is careful not to make judgments about the changing pace of life for kids, her study supports the impression that kids (and moms) are leading more hectic lives, with less time for pure play and family meals and conversation.

It's hard for parents to slow down and set appropriate limits on the family's expenditures of time and money, says Dr. Chambliss. Families with two working parents sometimes feel they have to buy the latest of everything and sign their kids up for every available activity to make up for the lack of time together, she explains. Sometimes, she says, it's easier to buy another new computer or let kids play another sport than to expend the emotional energy explaining why it's not necessary—or not going to improve their lives. In families with a single breadwinner, parents may feel apologetic about their lack of wealth and make unreasonable personal sacrifices in order to keep up with their neighbors.

Slow down and make sure your priorities are in the right order. Ask yourself these questions.

Are you doing what's important to you? Many women who come to Ruth Klein, a clinical psychologist and owner of The Marketing Time Source, say their families are important, but their schedules tell another story. They are rarely home, and when they are home, everyone is so busy running in different directions that there is no family time.

"What you role-model is what others perceive is important to you," Klein says. Her three children always knew their activities were important to her because of the time she spent attending their soccer, tennis, and volleyball games and their theater performances. Similarly, her family's nutrition and health are important, so she spends time shopping for and preparing healthy foods. Conversely,

Klein preserves time for her family and herself by paying $10 for a courier service to deliver packages across town or $16 to hire a college student to assist with the family dinner on Friday evenings. The student arrives near the end of dinner, makes coffee, serves dessert, and cleans the dishes and kitchen floor—while Mom enjoys her family.

Are you doing too much? You need to periodically appraise your family's extracurricular activities. If your son is crazy about a particular sport, group, or lesson and you like socializing at the events, it may be worth the time. But if he's ambivalent and you resent the effort, it may be time to drop it. Even if he likes the activities, you need to establish priorities.

Why are you doing this activity? Don't assume that just because the neighbor's child is participating in three activities, those three things will be good for your child. An introverted child may need more time to herself to explore the world in her own way.

Further, don't take on the responsibility for exploring these questions alone, says Dr. Sanik. "It's everybody's job to be a happy, well-adjusted family," she says. "Everybody needs to work on prioritizing and doing what's important."

Even if you set a rule, as many parents do, of one extracurricular activity at a time per child, if you have three children, things are still going to be pretty hectic—especially when you add chores, schoolwork, birthday parties, and get-togethers with friends. To help with the chaos, try establishing planning sheets just for the kids. These include each child's weekly household chores, sports and other lessons, social activities, and any recurring or big school projects. File them in your hanging file or a family organizer notebook. Then, when a child asks to add something to her schedule, tell her to check her planning sheets. It breeds an atmosphere of family cooperation and mutual responsibility, Schofield says.

Transitioning between Shifts

If you think "evening rush hour" describes the drive home, you haven't entered a house with kids just before dinnertime.

But before we get to the food part, we need to focus on the relaxation part. And it should start before we set foot in the house.

Use your drive time. On the ride home from work, don't fret about traffic or what went wrong with your day. Instead, think ahead to how you can organize your evening and carve out a niche for yourself. Decide what you can accomplish that evening, and promise yourself that when it's done, you'll relax.

Delay dinner. "Most moms think that as soon as they get home from work, they need to produce great meals for their families," says Alice D. Domar, Ph.D., a Harvard Medical School psychologist and director of the Mind/Body Center for Women's Health, Mind/Body Institute in Boston. "The last thing you need to do is walk in and start cooking." Take a breather. It may be 5 minutes in a quiet place; a 30-minute walk alone or with your dog, spouse, or kids; a glass of wine; or a quick nap in a hammock. It should be something to get you out of your work mode and ready to reconnect with your family in a relaxed way. After a quick, healthy snack, the children can wait a few minutes for dinner.

Focus on what's good. On average 70 percent of what happens to us each day is neutral, 15 percent is positive, and 15 percent is negative, but we tend to focus on the bad, says Dr. Domar, author of *Self-Nurture: Learning to Care for Yourself As Effectively As You Care for Everyone Else*. For example, when she walks through the door in the evening, Dr. Domar asks those who are there to tell her what happened new or good in their day. The "New and Good" game forces people to look at their day in a different way.

Create a sacred space. You need a place to sit and calm yourself, a place to shift out of the stress of ordinary activities and get back to yourself, says Judith Orloff, M.D., a Los Angeles psychiatrist and author of *Dr. Judith Orloff's Guide to Intuitive Healing: Five Steps to Physical, Emotional, and Sexual Wellness*, who lectures on the interrelationship

Dinner in a Flash

These dinners can be prepared in about 20 minutes, using canned, frozen, or otherwise partially prepared products.

Sunday: Grilled pork loin chops with packaged spice rub or marinade (cook enough for leftovers), quick-cooking couscous, and grilled asparagus seasoned with salt, pepper, olive oil, and lemon

Monday: Leftover pork thinly sliced atop a salad made from bagged greens, sun-dried tomatoes, and vinaigrette dressing

Tuesday: Pasta with packaged chopped chicken, broccoli florets, and pine nuts in a sauce made from canned chicken broth, topped with grated Parmesan

Wednesday: Use the leftover pasta (chicken, broccoli, and all) to create a frittata, mixing it with eggs, milk, and more Parmesan and cooking in a frying pan until firm.

Thursday: Frozen shrimp, frozen Oriental vegetables, and bottled sauce combined into a stir-fry and served with instant rice

Friday: Let the kids throw some toppings on a prepared pizza crust.

Saturday: Pan-seared sesame-encrusted salmon, Japanese udon noodles, and a fruit salad, using seasonal fruits and some of the salad greens and vinaigrette from Monday

of medicine, intuition, and spirituality. It may be a table with a candle, an incense holder, flowers, a bowl of fruit, or other favorite objects, or it may be as elaborate as an altar. It should be a place that's all your own, away from the hustle and bustle of the household. When you get home from work, spend at least 5 minutes there, just sitting and breathing.

Better Ways to Manage Mealtime

Most experts agree that eating dinner together strengthens the family. Early on, it's important to teach young children table manners and to instill family values and rituals, but the lessons and benefits don't end there. Communication is one of the main ingredients of the family meal, and it's also a key to raising emotionally healthy children, according to the National Safety Council. Ticklish topics—such as peer pressure and schoolwork—are more easily approached across the dinner table.

One study found that teenagers categorized as well-adjusted ate with their families an average of 5 days a week, while poorly adjusted teens ate with their families only 3 days a week.

The study didn't discover just what it is about family meals that helps teens deal with the pressures of adolescence—just that they seem to. If your family rarely has meals together, think about clearing some time.

Coordinate schedules to keep several nights a week clear, and if you can't clear enough nights, try breakfast some days. (But it doesn't count if you keep your nose in the newspaper or eyes on the television.)

Having family meals does require planning. And at 4 P.M. every day, 60 percent of us still have no idea what we're fixing for dinner. The key is planning ahead.

Make a list. Once a month, list your family's 15 favorite (and easiest) meals, shop for the ingredients, and put them in a designated place where they won't be gobbled up before you need them. Then post a list of menus on the inside of a cupboard door, and each morning, decide what to make that day, depending on what's going on with the family. Set out the recipe, and whoever gets home first starts dinner. Or post the week's plan on the refrigerator.

Delegate, delegate, delegate. Assign each member of the family (depending on age and ability) a particular night to cook. No complaining, however, if the cook doesn't have a green vegetable or if he serves the same thing every week.

Retire the short-order cook. Too many of us fall into the trap of cooking different meals for everyone in the family. We spend all night preparing, serving, and cleaning up food to accommodate various tastes and schedules. If someone must miss a meal or refuses to eat what's served, let her fend for herself—that's why microwaves were invented.

Have the basics. In addition to such staples as cooking oils, vinegars, sugar, flours, canned milk, herbs, and spices, your pantry might include such things as pastas, sun-dried tomatoes, canned tomatoes, tuna, anchovies, olives, chickpeas and other beans, salsa, refried beans, taco kits, rice, soy sauce, hoisin sauce, plum sauce, bean sprouts, and water chestnuts. Freezer standbys include frozen vegetables such as green beans, corn, peas, and spinach; pita bread; butter; frozen waffles; ginger (simply slice off a frozen piece); bags of chopped onions and peppers; packaged, deboned chicken breasts, sausages and bacon, and other meats; and extra cheeses.

Prepare as you put away. Just back from the grocery store? Before you stash that ground meat in the freezer, toss it into a frying pan and brown it; then freeze it for quick additions to spaghetti sauce or casseroles. Wash salad greens and store them in a plastic bag in the refrigerator; grate cheese and freeze in bulk; chop some onions and green peppers and freeze in plastic bags; and clean and cut up veggies and fruit for snacks and lunches.

Think double. It takes about 6 minutes to throw together one meat loaf; it takes 7 minutes to make three. With just an extra minute, you have two meals in the freezer. Dovetail processes as well as dishes, such as using the food processor to shred cheese for tonight's tacos, cabbage for tomorrow's coleslaw, and carrots for vegetable meatballs.

Cook for leftovers. Roast two or three chickens at one time. After the first night, use leftovers in chicken curry; tossed with pasta and broccoli; on an open-faced sandwich with avocado and tomato; in quesadillas or burritos; and mixed with vegetables for a quick frittata or omelette. Similarly, a large batch of meat loaf does yeoman's duty as the makings for meatball stroganoff, stuffed grape leaves, and meat loaf sandwiches. Even extra mashed potatoes can be recycled—into potato puffs, potato pancakes, or shepherd's pie—or used as a thickener for soups and sauces.

Make it snappy. Don't hesitate to use prepared or partially prepared foods to make life easier. There are lots of high-quality convenience products out there, including bags of vegetables that need only the addition of some ground turkey to make a nutritious stir-fry.

Never run out. Always have a running shopping list accessible to the whole family. It's even more efficient to have one set up by categories. Schofield suggests these categories: breads and cereals, canned goods, convenience foods, dairy and eggs, frozen foods, health and beauty aids, household and miscellaneous, meat, produce, and staples and condiments. To take it a step further, organize your list according to your grocery store's layout; many stores will give you a guide.

Shop smart. Buy two of such nonperishable items as toothpaste, shampoo, and detergent. When the first one runs out, add the item to the shopping list; this saves emergency runs to the store.

When It's Time to Pay

If you've delegated, decluttered, and organized but you're still dragging, maybe it's time to hire help. "It's the way to go in two regards," says Dr. Chambliss. "First, you're liberating time for more important activities. And it can help you detach a little from the whole emotional issue. If you get outside help, it's no longer your thing."

Decide which chores you'd most like to dump—and do so. Hire a housekeeper, a gardener, a cook, a courier service, a chef, a caregiver—or a college student. Even if you can't afford a weekly housekeeper, it'll give you a big energy boost to hire a couple of college students to help with the annual spring cleaning.

There are many professional organizations geared toward personal needs, such as the National Association of Professional Organizers. For an hourly fee, a pro will help you sort through the clutter that has become your life and get you started on a new, less time-consuming track. (Call 512-206-0151 or visit the association's Web site at www.napo.net.)

Similarly, the United States Personal Chef Association provides another fast-growing profession. With a click or a phone call, you can hire a personal chef who will buy groceries and come to your home once a week or so and fix meals to your liking, to be frozen and thawed when you need them. The chef will even freeze individual portions for families where everyone eats on a different schedule. Call (800) 995-2138 or visit the association's Web sites at www.uspca.com and www.hireachef.com.

Low on cash? Swap meals with a neighbor, organize car pools, even grab a friend and take turns cleaning each other's house as a team—the work will go faster and be more fun.

And fun, after all, should be part of life on the home front. "If you're not having any fun, find some," says Dr. Schenkel.

Relationships: Turning Sappers into Sustainers

As Ben climbs into bed, Carolyn rolls the other way, her back toward him. "Not tonight," she thinks. It's a familiar feeling. Sex is the furthest thing from her mind most nights. She feels guilty over her lack of desire and sad for the loss of passion in their relationship, but although she still loves Ben, these days sex seems like just one more item on her increasingly long to-do list.

There's no question that the care and feeding of the people in our lives require a tremendous amount of time and energy. Too often, we focus on meeting everyone else's expectations and ignore our own, leaving ourselves spent and depleted. Yet if we learn how to balance what we give with what we get from our relationships, the people in our lives may actually turn into energy sustainers instead of energy sappers.

"Relationships can be extremely energizing if there is mutuality, if we *allow* them to be two-way rather than try to be the source of all giving," says Maria M. Mancusi, Ph.D., a clinical psychologist from Springfield, Virginia.

Five Things That Sap Your Energy

While men are defined more by their achievements, women are defined by their relationships. Helping others and being available to listen and provide support are central roles in our lives.

Think you're immune? Jot down all the roles you fill during an average week—wife, mother, daughter, friend, employee, chauffeur, tutor, housewife, boss, neighbor, church volunteer, social coordinator. The list goes on.

"There's a big debate about how all these relationships affect our energy levels," says Simone Ravicz, Ph.D., a psychologist in Pacific Palisades, California, and author of *High on Stress: A Woman's Guide to Optimizing the Stress in Her Life*. Some experts believe that we have a limited amount of energy and that the more roles we occupy in life, the less energy we have. It's a concept psychologists call the *scarcity theory*.

Dr. Ravicz, however, has another view. Tackling multiple roles boosts our self-esteem, while a strong social support network actually *increases* our energy levels—a theory called the *enhancement hypothesis*.

"The mere fact that you have several roles doesn't mean you'll suffer from less energy," says Dr. Ravicz.

It's a hard concept to grasp, especially since so many of us feel like a limp dishrag by the end of the day. The difference, says Dr. Ravicz, is how many energy drainers we've integrated into our roles and relationships. They include the following:

Stress. Studies show that while men stress out over infrequent events like loss of income, we stress out over everyday events that involve those close to us. We worry about our best friend's divorce, stew over an unreasonable request from the boss, or wonder how long an ailing parent will be able to manage independently. All this mental caretaking drives up stress levels, wearing us out physically and mentally.

Too much give, too little take. People drain us when all they do is make demands of us, yet we don't feel free to ask for something in return. "Women are socialized to give, give, give," says Dr. Ravicz. "Our socialization has trained us to feel obligated to be responsive to others' needs, even at the cost of our own. We're not socialized to draw boundaries, so we end up giving too much." The irony is that by spreading ourselves so thin, we often end up disappointing the very people we're trying to please. And because of social conditioning, we feel guilty when we're the ones reaching out for support.

The answer, says Dr. Ravicz, is to remember that healthy, life-sustaining relationships are a two-way deal.

Lack of intimacy. Ironically, a lack of intimate relationships can be just as draining as a plethora of them, says Sandra Haber, Ph.D., a New York City psychologist who specializes in women's issues. Intimate relationships help balance our emotional bank account by giving us time to just be ourselves. They are the few special relationships in our lives in which we feel comfortable seeking out as much support as we give. "When we spend all of our time tending to superficial relationships, we spend too much time with our masks on, and there's no time to be authentic," says Dr. Haber.

Biting our proverbial tongue. The minute we start denying, repressing, or suppressing our feelings to those we're involved with, we drain our energy. It's like driving a car with one foot on the accelerator and the other on the brakes. "If you don't express how you feel, you wind up covering up the feeling, and that takes energy," says Dr. Haber.

Suppose your husband asks if you'd mind having a colleague for dinner tomorrow night. You think to yourself, "No way! I have such a long day tomorrow. I don't want to do it." But instead you say, "Oh, sure."

As women, we're socialized to be "nice." So we go along with a request even if it makes us angry, uncomfortable, or resentful. By not voicing how we feel, we limit our options, explains Dr. Haber. If you say to your husband, "Tomorrow's a busy day for me; I don't know if I can do this," then the two of you can work out a compromise—perhaps go out for dinner or schedule it on another night.

Parenting a Teenager Is Exhausting

Here's how to survive the teen years without taking to your bed, says Maria M. Mancusi, Ph.D., a clinical psychologist in Springfield, Virginia.

Pick your battles. Take stands on the important issues, not trivial ones. You'll have a much better chance of success.

Be consistent. Develop a set of family values and stick to them—a curfew, study time, relationships with siblings. When these values are challenged, be consistent in how you deal with it.

Reinforce the positive. Emphasize your teen's triumphs—big or small. Some parents show emotion only when their adolescent misbehaves. It's important to spontaneously comment on something your teenager does that you appreciate.

Minimize the negative. Don't overreact. Limit your response when you're angry, and move on. Don't say things you'll regret later.

Keep score. Start a diary in which you log each problem and argument, including what set off the episode, how long it lasted, and what helped. Instead of worrying about how it makes you feel, concentrate on what is actually happening.

Not spending enough time alone. The most important relationship is the one you have with yourself. An hour or even a half-hour of leisure each day is necessary for refueling your energy, not a reward for completing all your tasks. This should be quality time—taking a walk, meditating, reading, or even soaking in a hot bath. As long as you enjoy it, it's energizing, says Dr. Haber. The key is to plan for it, not just to wait for free time to appear.

Energizing Your Relationships

Nothing is more energy draining than trying to change another person's behavior. So the path to energizing relationships is more a matter of shifting your own perceptions, reevaluating your own expectations, or redefining the way you communicate with others.

"It's an American myth that you should always tell others when you're upset with them to try to get them to change," notes Karen Fingerman, Ph.D., assistant professor of human development at Pennsylvania State University in State College. "That may be good advice for some married couples, for example, but not for every relationship." Instead, you need to focus on changing how you perceive or react to the other person.

By making one positive change in each of the following relationships, you can get what you want: more energy.

With Your Mother

Agree to disagree. Accepting Mom for who she is seems to be the key to easing mother–daughter tensions, according to Dr. Fingerman's research. She's found that in the most positive mother–daughter relationships, the daughter is able to view Mom's annoying traits as simply those—annoying traits—not deliberate acts designed to drive her crazy.

"Daughters who are able to say 'That's how Mom is' or 'That's just her way' fare best," Dr. Fingerman says. On the other hand, when a daughter perceives her mother's attention as an intrusion or as critical in some way, the relationship suffers.

Acceptance is a matter of shifting your perception of the situation, she says. For example, maybe your mother has lousy taste in clothes. When you open the baby clothes she bought, you can either view her gift as her foisting her taste on your kids when she knows full well that's not what you want them to wear or laugh about it and chalk it up to a simple flaw in your mother.

It helps to understand that part of the reason you see things differently from your mother is because each of you is at a different point in your life, Dr. Fingerman says. The good news, however, is that research shows your relationship with Mom actually improves as you age.

With Your Friends

Lean on them. Research shows that friends—not partners—are often your best source of emotional support. While men are apt to name their spouses or girlfriends as their main source of support, women are more likely to name another woman, usually a friend, sister, or mother, explains Susan Lynch, Ph.D., director of the bachelor of social work program at the University of Arkansas at Little Rock.

The problem is we tend to be more comfortable *giving* support than getting it, even with our friends. For us, reciprocity is a big issue. When we get something from a friend, our comfort level goes way down, Dr. Lynch says, and we want to pay back the favor quickly. So when we're

Falling in Love Again

"You can fall out of love just as easily as you fall in love," says Marilyn Fithian, Ph.D., a licensed marriage and family counselor in Long Beach, California. "The most important thing is to decide what love is to you."

Look beyond passion. "Friendship is the crucial element," Dr. Fithian says. "Without a genuine enjoyment of spending time together, there's not much point to any relationship." Since even the best relationships can get stale, try these approaches.

Separating. Just temporarily! Take a vacation away from him. "Sometimes you don't know how much a relationship means until you miss your partner for a while," she says.

Surprises. Arrange a surprise trip for just the two of you. Have the bags packed and the kids camped elsewhere

overburdened, we avoid unloading on friends because we're not sure we can reciprocate. We're afraid they'll say, "All Susan does is gripe."

"Give yourself permission to need support," Dr. Lynch says. "Cultivate your friendships with women. They tend to be the least demanding and the most supportive of relationships, yet they're the first thing we cut from our busy lives." Best bet: Seek out friends you can share a laugh with. The most energizing friendships are *fun friendships*.

With Your Partner

Rekindle the flame. Nearly one in three women between the ages of 30 and 60 isn't interested in sex, according to the National Health and Social Life Survey, a study of sexual behavior in American adults. It's a sure bet

when he gets home from work. "Sometimes all you need to do is go to the motel across town," says Dr. Fithian.

Touching. Dr. Fithian often uses caress exercises with couples in crisis. "This usually goes on for 2 or 3 hours—touching, kissing, hugging, patting."

Sharing. Maybe you're not big into sports, but he is. Or you hate fishing. Once in a while, ask to tag along. "Your partner will appreciate the effort and be more inclined to get involved in something you really enjoy," says Dr. Fithian.

Relaxing. Take a walk around the neighborhood or go out for ice cream. "Do some of the simple things you did together before you got married," she says. "And take your time with these things, which have always spawned communication naturally."

that a chronic lack of energy is part of the problem. So is the fact that when two people have been together for a long time, sex can get dull.

The solution? "Touching does a lot in terms of adding energy to a relationship," says Marilyn Fithian, Ph.D., codirector for the Marital & Sexual Studies Work in Long Beach, California. "It adds spark back into a marriage." By taking the time more often to caress, hug, and kiss, she says, you can restore the passion and energy in your relationship.

To help her clients reconnect emotionally, physically, and spiritually with their partners, Dr. Fithian prescribes a touch exercise she calls "caress therapy." When they begin, couples spend 30 to 60 minutes simply touching and caressing each other's hands, face, and feet (set a timer if you need to). You can use massage oil, but make sure you pick it out together.

Couples gradually work up to a 2- to 3-hour exercise. "We've had couples holed up in a room for an entire weekend doing caress exercises but never having intercourse," Dr. Fithian says. "It meant so much more in terms of being in love. The goal here isn't sexual. It's a great way to discover each other again on a very personal level."

With People at Work

Keep it positive. Negative people drain energy. Listening to a coworker whine about her workload, her manager, or her working conditions is a real downer, says Filomena Warihay, Ph.D., president of Take Charge Consultants, an international management training and organizational development firm in Downingtown, Pennsylvania. Often you'll try to help by offering a solution, but the whiner responds with an objection. You offer another suggestion, and the whiner retorts with another "Yeah, but . . ."

"The downward spiral continues until you are exhausted, and the whiner starts whining about you and your inability to understand or be helpful," says Dr. Warihay. A surefire way to avoid the whiner and keep your workday energized: Ask a couple of questions. "What would you like to have happen instead?" And "What are you going to do to get what you need?"

Overall, says Dr. Ravicz, "relationships can wear us out, but they are also what get us through our day-to-day crises. Self-management and balance are the name of the game."

And balance starts by learning to set boundaries. To establish a comfort zone, you need to know what you are willing to do *and* what you're not willing to do. The most important thing we can learn, she says, is how to say no when we're stretched too thin.

Thriving in the
Sandwich Generation

The sun warms Carolyn's face as she steps outside. *It's going to be a beautiful Saturday*, she says to herself. *Too bad I'll be cleaning Mother's house all day.*

As she drives to her mother's house, Carolyn thinks about the challenges of the past year, how her 79-year-old mother's arthritis has become so severe the older woman can no longer cook or clean. Even getting dressed has become a chore, especially if there are buttons to be fastened.

Enter Superdaughter.

Giving up what little free time she has, Carolyn has begun cleaning her mother's house, paying the bills, and taking dinner to her most days. But lately it doesn't seem to be enough. Sometimes when Carolyn stops by after work, her mother is still wearing a bathrobe.

Even worse, her mother's health problems are multiplying. The arthritis is getting worse, and the doctor just diagnosed her with hypertension, prescribing even more drugs.

Lately, Carolyn's been thinking about an assisted living facility for her mother, where someone can help with everyday activities like dressing and bathing. But every time she's about to bring it up, an overwhelming sense of sadness and guilt silences her. This woman, who never completed college, managed to raise three children on a secretary's salary when her husband died at 34. Now, to see her unable to even tie her own shoes breaks Carolyn's heart. If she sent her mother to a home, she'd feel like she was turning her back on her.

So Carolyn's simply added the job of caregiver to her already crowded résumé.

When Enough Is Enough

There's going to be a day when Mom requires much more than you, your relatives, or your friends can handle. But admitting you can't do it all doesn't mean turning her over to the care of strangers. Many options short of a nursing home exist.

Adult day care. These centers offer services for older adults who've had strokes, paralysis, or early dementia or who are in wheelchairs. Fees, around $70 a day, are often charged on a sliding-scale basis. The staff provides a variety of services, including crafts, exercises, minimal medical care, and bathing. Trained nurses are available to give medications.

Home health care. You could have a skilled nurse, capable of providing medical treatment, come to your home once a day for about $70. If Mom's needs are the result of hospitalization, the cost may be covered by Medicare. A home-care aide, who provides personal assistance with dressing, bathing, and feeding, may cost $10 to $18 an hour.

Assisted living facility. This type of facility provides 24-hour services but offers far more independence than a nursing home. Mom gets help with personal care, from

Carolyn's situation is far from unique, and the way things are going in this country, it's going to become far more common.

The number of people age 65 and older is expected to grow to 20 percent of the population by the year 2030. Our parents—often our mothers because women live longer than men—are also living longer and remaining at home instead of moving into nursing homes. Today, 23 percent of households contain at least one person who is

bathing to receiving hot meals, in an apartment-like setting. "The biggest reason people move into assisted living is because they need help taking their medication," says Elinor Ginzler, a spokesperson for AARP in Washington, D.C. Costs could range from $1,000 to $4,000 a month and are rarely covered by insurance.

Board and care. These facilities typically offer many of the amenities of an assisted living facility but in a smaller, more homelike atmosphere, often in someone's private home. Costs range from $350 to $3,000 a month and are rarely covered by insurance. For information, contact your local office on aging (usually listed in the blue pages of the phone book) or EldercareLocator (800-677-1116).

For help with a parent who doesn't live near you, try a geriatric care manager. You can find one through the Eldercare Locator or through the National Association of Geriatric Care Managers at www.caremanager.org. Fees vary from $50 to $100 for the initial consultation. Be a smart consumer, Ginzler says, by pricing several managers and making sure they have either a background in nursing, with geriatrics experience, or a master's degree in social work.

caring for an older relative or friend. And 73 percent of those caregivers are women.

Why We Do It All

"There's an expectation that women will do it and that they're more comfortable and experienced doing the job," says Ramsey McGowen, Ph.D., associate professor in the department of psychiatry and behavioral sciences at East Tennessee State University in Johnson City. But before you go around blaming men, consider our own complicity in this. After all, if we didn't still buy into the old stereotype about "women's work," would we still be the ones doing most of the housework and child care?

Gender isn't the only factor. "Almost invariably there's a caregiver in families," says Barbara Ensor, Ph.D., a psychologist at the geriatric facility at Stella Maris in Baltimore. "You can pick them out when they're children." They're the babysitters, the ones making dinner every night, those supervising bath time.

Then there's guilt. Our parents did so much for us for so long, making so many sacrifices; now it's our turn. We should put *them* before anything else, the way they put *us* before anything else. It's a role reversal.

The Job Itself

Caring for a parent is like adding a full-time job to your life. Many caregivers spend 20 or more hours each week in the role, doing everything from dusting to driving to opening mail.

Forget the obvious result—exhaustion. We're also talking major health problems. You know the old saying "Who cares for the caregiver?" Usually, no one.

For instance, a National Family Caregivers Association survey found that caregivers experienced more headaches, stomach problems, back pain, sleeplessness, and depression than before they began the role. The problems weren't limited to physical health. Episodes of frustration, anxiety, and sadness also increased.

And this is for the long haul, says Mary Pipher, Ph.D., a psychologist and the author of *Another Country: Navigating the Emotional Terrain of Our Elders*. We might be able to care for Mom around the clock when she's got 6 weeks left to live, but we'll never keep up that frenzied pace for 5, 10, or 20 years. "Some people get burned-out at the very point when their parent is in desperate need," she says.

Not only do our extra responsibilities cut into family and free time, but also they often disrupt the hours we spend at work. Half of all caregivers who are employed have to change their work schedules—going in late, leaving early, or taking time off in the middle of the day. While some companies give time off, many people must use their own vacation time or cut their hours at work.

Also, little chores for our parents turn into big projects. When we want to make a fast trip to the store, Mom wants to stop for coffee and a bite to eat (which she nibbles at for an hour). We want to drop off some dinner and sprint to our son's soccer game, but Dad has a list of chores he needs completed *now*.

Then there are the age-old parent–child issues.

If Mom never worked outside the home, she might have no idea how stressful it is to commute or what it's like to report to a boss every day and still try to be a supermom. And if you're caregiver to your father, who never washed a plate or cooked a meal in his life, he's not going to have a clue about your second shift.

So you need to do some educating. Talk about your frustrations at work, laugh about the difficulties of raising kids, and be open about your day-to-day activities, Dr. Ensor suggests. This will help your parents understand you better and make your job as caregiver easier.

Sleep Habits Change As We Age

The older you are, the lighter your sleep. It's a gradual process that begins around age 20 and seems to be part of normal aging. There are several reasons for the change.

You're more prone to sleep disorders, such as sleep apnea and restless legs syndrome, as you age. This is due to reduced REM sleep, the sleep time in which you dream; increased sensitivity to your sleeping environment; less efficient sleep; and a host of other factors. And the internal clock that tells you when to go to sleep and when to wake up seems to slip forward, making you feel sleepy earlier in the evening and waking you earlier.

Researchers think these changes might be related to a decrease in growth hormone production, which is secreted during deep sleep, and melatonin, a hormone that helps us sleep. Medical problems such as arthritis, heartburn, osteoporosis, and heart and lung disease, along with the medications that treat them, also keep us from sleeping well.

The good news: The healthier you are, the better you snooze.

"Generally, very healthy people have no problems with their sleep, no matter what their age," says Sonia Ancoli-Israel, Ph.D., a psychiatry professor at the University of California, San Diego, and author of *All I Want Is a Good Night's Sleep*.

But remember the Golden Rule of the Adult Child: You can't tell your parents what to do. "That just doesn't work," Ensor says. "They are still the parents."

A 7-Step Prevention Plan

What you *can* do is give Mom as much control of her life as possible. If someone else has to handle your mother's finances, for example, let her decide who does it if she can. If Dad is going into an assisted living facility, take him on the tours with you so he can ask questions. Let him make choices, such as whether he'd like a room by the kitchen or by the garden. If you're hiring a home health aide, let your mother interview the best two and choose one.

Still, like parenting, this is a job that only gets tougher, so you've got to keep an eye peeled for burnout. Experts say you're doing too much if:

- You haven't talked to a friend in 2 weeks.
- You haven't gone out socially in at least a week.
- You're getting less than 7 hours of sleep a night.
- You're getting sick more often than usual.
- You're smoking or drinking more than usual.
- You don't have the energy to talk about your stress.
- You can't concentrate, whether it's to read a book, balance your checkbook, or follow a recipe.
- You're more forgetful than usual.
- You're missing out on things you really want to do, such as going to your kids' baseball games.
- You're more irritable than usual.
- You start to think Mom is faking her symptoms.

If you recognize yourself in any of these symptoms, you're in desperate need of the one thing caregivers most lust after: time for yourself. You need the Caregiver-in-Control Plan. Here's how it works.

Step 1. Lay out your own life. Take a daily calendar and fill in the days and hours with everything you do outside of caregiving: work, cooking, chauffeuring, laundry, cleaning, shopping, bill paying. And don't forget to schedule yourself in. Whether it's an hour every day or an entire evening every week to take a bubble bath, read a book, or watch your favorite television show, you deserve it.

Step 2. Lay out Mom's life. List everything that needs to be done for your parent and see what you can reasonably fit into your schedule, such as having Mom over for dinner three times a week and doing her laundry on Wednesdays.

Step 3. Show Mom. When she sees your schedule on paper, she'll realize just how frantic your life really is. It will provide a blast of reality and maybe help assuage some of your own guilt, says Dr. McGowen. Even if Mom is too sick to understand, seeing all this on paper will make it clearer to *you* that you can't make dinner, clean the house, do three loads of laundry, and check on Mom in the 1 hour between work and dinner.

Step 4. Call a meeting. Gather Mom, husband, kids, relatives, and any neighbors and friends willing to help. Make sure they understand the seriousness of the situation and where it's going in the future. Bring pamphlets and medical records (with Mom's permission) to update them on her health. Then show them your schedule so they, too, understand just what the term *Superdaughter* really means. Sure, you're pawning some of the guilt off on them, but if that makes it harder for them to turn down your plea for help next time, it's worth it.

Step 5. Brainstorm solutions. Some ideas:

- Hire a maid (for you or for Mom).
- Assign duties to the kids. They can cut the grass, read to Grandma, or even take her to doctors' appointments if they're old enough.
- Use a transportation service specifically for older adults.
- Hire a teenager to mow Mom's lawn or do her grocery shopping.
- Sign up for a Meals on Wheels program to deliver hot meals.
- Ask out-of-town relatives to visit for a week to give you a break. Or set up a time for your parent to visit them. If they don't have the time but want to help out, suggest that they chip in for laundry or maid service.
- Suggest jobs that match a relative's own strengths and weaknesses. If your sister can't be in the same room with Mom without fighting, assign her the bills to pay so she and Mom don't have to talk.
- Keep your parents active and help them find their own circle of support. Look for activities at your local senior citizens center and volunteer opportunities at libraries, hospitals, and schools. Perhaps they would enjoy exercise classes specifically for their age group. The busier they are, the more in control and happier they'll be.

Step 6. Maintain. Don't stop after one meeting. The core group of people who have agreed to care for Mom should meet at least every 2 weeks in the beginning to keep the lines of communication open. You might want to rotate responsibilities after a few weeks.

Step 7. Seek support. While you're at it, sign yourself up for a support group. "People don't understand that one of the reasons we're so busy is because we're trying to do everything ourselves," Dr. Pipher says. But building a community of people who support you saves time and energy. You'll find resources through other members, and you

Where to Get Help

There's an entire world of people out there willing to help caregivers, sometimes on a volunteer basis.

- The National Association of Area Agencies on Aging provides the EldercareLocator, which helps identify nationwide information and referral services to help with care for the aged (800-677-1116 or www.n4a.org).
- National Institute on Aging (www.nih.gov/nia)
- American Association of Retired Persons (www.aarp.org)
- National Association for Home Care (www.nahc.org)
- American Association of Homes and Services for the Aging (www.aahsa.org)
- Alzheimer's Association (www.alz.org)
- National Family Caregivers Association (www.nfcacares.org)
- National Alliance for Caregiving (www.caregiving.org)
- Other local charities and organizations you could contact include United Way, Family Services of America, Jewish Family Services, Catholic Charities, Protestant Welfare Agencies, the American Red Cross, the Visiting Nurses Association, social service agencies, and local churches. For organizations in your area, check your phone book.

might find companions for your parent. But most important, you'll be able to talk to a group of people who know exactly what you're going through. Look for information at community centers or your place of worship.

Once Carolyn joined a support group, her life was transformed. She met a woman whose mother lives in an assisted living facility that she adores. Carolyn was able to introduce her mother to the older woman and suggest that she think about moving into the same facility. Her mother agreed. Now that the facility does Mom's laundry and cooks her meals, Carolyn has more time to just *be* with her mother, going to movies, taking walks, or simply sitting and talking.

When Illness Is the Culprit

Carolyn sighs as she hangs up the phone. Her friend Marcia, a collegiate partner-in-crime and fellow soccer mom, has chronic fatigue syndrome (CFS). She had a really bad day today after spending the weekend at a soccer tournament. The games are over, but Marcia's day-after pain has just begun—worse than any New Year's Day hangover.

"Why do I always do this to myself?" Marcia asked Carolyn in a voice so weak Carolyn had to strain to hear. "Why can't I just take it easy like my doctors recommend?"

"Because you've never taken it easy," Carolyn answered honestly, thinking of Marcia's nonstop energy in college. Her friend would stay up all night preparing a presentation or writing a paper, only to spend the next night dancing until dawn. After college, Marcia worked full-time and went to business school, simultaneously earning promotions and her M.B.A. in record time. Was it any wonder "relaxing" wasn't in her vocabulary?

Then Marcia's doctor told her she had chronic fatigue

syndrome. Carolyn remembers her reaction when Marcia broke the news. "Chronic fatigue syndrome?" Carolyn scoffed aloud. "What woman with a husband, kids, job, and house *doesn't* have chronic fatigue syndrome?"

When to See a Doctor

Talk to your doctor if you answer yes to any of these questions.

- Are you too tired to manage activities of daily living, such as showering, cooking, cleaning, caring for your children, and working?
- Do you still feel exhausted even after a vacation?
- Are you habitually tired even when you should be well-rested?
- Are you still fighting off the flu or the cold everyone else in the office had—and recovered from—weeks ago?
- Did lifestyle changes (such as moving to a better climate for your allergies or eating a healthier diet) make no difference in your fatigue?
- Have you recently gained or lost 5 percent of your body weight without dieting or changing your habits?
- Do you have muscle aches and joint pains that just don't go away?
- Have you had fevers recently that you just couldn't explain?
- Do your hands or feet turn colors when they get cold?
- Have you been severely tired for 6 months or more?
- Have you had swollen glands for no apparent reason?
- Does it take you more than 24 hours to recover from physical exertion?

Years later she still cringes when she recalls that flip remark. CFS has proven to be a tough competitor for even an all-star like Marcia to beat. While she's gotten better, she still isn't at 100 percent and doesn't know if she ever will be again.

"Thankfully, there's nothing wrong with me that a good night's rest won't help," Carolyn thinks to herself as she pads upstairs to fold the laundry before bed.

Chronic Fatigue Syndrome

CFS represents a serious health problem that's difficult to diagnose and challenging to treat. Yet it's relatively benign compared with other health issues.

"The good news is, it won't shorten your life. It won't put you in a wheelchair. It won't lead to other problems," says Mary B. Duke, M.D., associate professor of internal medicine and pediatrics at the University of Kentucky in Lexington. And although there's no known cure for CFS, it's not an incurable disease. About half of CFS patients recover from the disorder, most of them within 5 years. Still, the disease is three times more common in women than men, affecting as many as 800,000 people each year.

For many women, CFS starts like "the flu from hell," says Dr. Duke. Except this flu never seems to go away, leaving you tired, weak, and spent after seemingly minor exertion. You may think you're just extraordinarily exhausted from finishing last month's big project at work, but sleep doesn't help either. Many CFS sufferers turn to exercise, telling themselves, "If I just work out, I'll get my energy back." But their efforts backfire, leaving them barely able to get out of bed the next day.

Other symptoms include the following.

- Memory and concentration problems
- Sore throat

- Unrefreshing sleep
- Tenderness in the lymph nodes, located in the neck, armpits, abdomen, and groin
- Muscle pain
- Joint pain without redness or swelling
- Headaches that vary in their severity or pattern compared with headaches you've had before

If you're experiencing any four of the above and you've been severely fatigued for 6 months or more, talk to your doctor about CFS. Be prepared for lots of tests: blood work, urinalysis, thyroid, even cognitive exams that ask about your concentration or memory. Before your doctor can diagnose you with CFS, she needs to rule out everything else that can cause fatigue, such as depression, sleep problems, and autoimmune diseases.

What's Happening?

No one really knows what causes CFS. Some speculate that extreme stress or viral infections, such as colds and the flu, may somehow spark the immune system into overdrive, leaving your body fighting as though you had a perpetual case of the flu.

Other theories suggest that the central nervous system is responsible since physical or emotional stress activates the hypothalamic–pituitary–adrenal gland axis, leading to the increased release of stress hormones.

Researchers are also looking at the role low blood pressure plays since both CFS patients and those with a condition known as neurally mediated hypotension (NMH) seem to experience dizziness, light-headedness, or fatigue after standing for a long time or in warm places. Researchers think drugs for NMH might help CFS patients as well.

Some suggest CFS may have connections to both our minds and our bodies—not just one or the other. According to one study, those with CFS reported more negative life events and infections before the syndrome's onset than those without. "This mind–body link makes sense intuitively," says Susan K. Johnson, Ph.D., assistant professor of psychology at the University of North Carolina at Charlotte. "But it's very hard for people to grasp that model."

Doctors need to acknowledge that CFS is a real disease, says Dr. Johnson, but patients also need to deal with the fact that their lifestyles or thought patterns, too, may be a contributing factor. "The connection of CFS with stress is a tricky one," she says. "Some studies show that people with CFS had a very active, high-stress lifestyle before they got sick." But such recollections are not reliable, she says, so the connection is still murky.

Finding Help for CFS

One of the single most important steps toward recovery is finding a doctor who believes you even *have* the disease. Sounds simple, but often it's not.

Validation may be more important in CFS than with other chronic illnesses precisely because it is less socially legitimate, according to Barbara Saltzstein, a Harvard Medical School psychiatry lecturer. She found that women with CFS who were diagnosed early and found a CFS-friendly physician who was optimistic about their future health were likelier to report more improvement than those who didn't.

If your doctor's a CFS skeptic, call a nearby medical school and ask if it has a CFS clinic. Rheumatologists, immunologists, and primary care physicians also treat CFS. Although there's no cure for CFS yet, there are several approaches, including the following:

Antidepressants. Prescribed in small doses, these medications (generally selective serotonin reuptake inhibitors, such as Prozac and the older, tricyclic drugs) help you sleep better. They may also ease the muscle and joint pain that troubles some CFS sufferers.

NADH. This substance helps the cells in our body produce energy—a process that's disrupted in CFS patients. In one study, 31 percent of those on the dietary supplement for 1 month felt better. Be aware that nervousness, loss of appetite, and stomach upset have been reported by some people in the first few days of supplementing. Follow label instructions for dosages.

Emotional therapy. A specific psychotherapy approach known as cognitive behavioral therapy (CBT) is helpful in coping with the emotional frustration of CFS. "This disease can be devastating to successful women who are used to performing and achieving—it's become part of their identities," says Dr. Duke. "But when all they can do in a day is walk to the mailbox and wash their hair, that doesn't feel like success. CBT helps them redefine what success is."

Exercise. As unappealing as it sounds when you feel perpetually exhausted, you need to move your muscles. Otherwise, both your cardiovascular system and your muscles will get weaker and weaker, making such everyday tasks as climbing stairs, carrying laundry, and even taking a shower that much harder. Dr. Duke suggests working into your day up to 30 minutes of low-impact aerobic exercise, such as walking and bicycling.

Relaxation. "Women with CFS tend to overdo it," says Billy Brennan, a mental health practitioner at Harborview Medical Center's Chronic Fatigue Clinic in Seattle. "When they're having a good day, they try to get as much done as possible." To guard against overexertion, keep a notebook in which you jot down your activities and look for connections. Were you worn-out on Thursday after 6 hours of shopping Wednesday but okay on Monday after only 3 hours of Sunday gardening? Maybe 3 hours is your physical limit.

Multivitamins. "They're not a cure," cautions Dr. Duke. "They're nutritional insurance because many of us don't eat right." Some researchers have suggested that people with CFS are deficient in magnesium or B vitamins, but Dr. Duke says that "hasn't panned out" for CFS patients as a group.

Support. A chronic health problem such as CFS can be socially isolating. Check your newspaper for support groups that can offer companionship and understanding.

Other Causes of Continual Fatigue

Not every woman's fatigue can be chalked up to a busy schedule and too little sleep. But neither is a bad case of exhaustion always something as serious as CFS.

"Most of the time, there are other explanations." says Dr. Duke. Springtime allergies can make us restless one moment and woozy the next, especially when we're popping decongestants and antihistamines. A bout with the flu can leave us prostrate on the couch for days.

Sometimes the culprit's even less obvious. "Sinus infections can be low-grade infections with vague symptoms," says Elizabeth Burns, M.D., professor of family medicine at the University of Illinois at Chicago. "People come in and say, 'I just don't feel right. I just don't have the energy I used to.'"

These concerns may sound minor, but their impact on our energy levels isn't. Fighting off an infection is a major undertaking for the body. When bacteria or a virus appears in the bloodstream, cells known as lymphocytes start making antibodies, disease-fighting molecules that recognize and match the unique proteins of the bacteria or virus. Those antibodies go into the bloodstream and attack the invader.

In the process, body temperature rises in response to inflammatory chemicals that reset the internal thermostat. We're hot to the touch, yet we get the chills as our muscles try to warm up to our new, higher body temperature. We feel exhausted because the energy we might normally use for exercising, concentrating at work, or making dinner is being diverted to battle the virus. If it's an invader we haven't seen before, prepare for bodily combat.

"When your body's being challenged by a virus your system's never seen, the virus builds up in numbers before your immune system has the antibodies to fight it off— and you are one sick puppy," says Dr. Burns.

Allergies may not be as dramatic, but they're just as unpleasant. Between the congestion, the postnasal drip, the snoring from a stuffed-up nose, and the sometimes stimulating, sometimes sedating side effects of the medications we're taking, sleep is darn hard to come by. No wonder we sleepwalk through the day when pollen counts are high.

There are multiple ways to beat energy busters like colds, allergies, and the flu.

Pick simple medications. If allergy or cold medicines leave you hyped up at night, look for a simple antihistamine (such as Benadryl) to take before sleeping; it tends to be more sedating. If drowsiness is your problem, choose a decongestant, which is generally more stimulating, although it can cause sleepiness in some people. Follow package instructions for dosage. Talk to your doctor if over-the-counter drugs don't work for you; newer prescription medications, such as Allegra and Claritin, may have less dramatic side effects, says Dr. Burns.

Take long, hot showers. When nasal passages are blocked as a result of a cold, allergies, or a sinus infection, the steam and moisture of showering often help them drain.

Fatigue in Early Pregnancy

Hormones probably play a role in the fatigue many women experience in the early months of pregnancy. It's not all in your head.

During the first 3 months, there's a major increase in two hormones: human chorionic gonadotropin (hCG) and progesterone. When women use products that contain progesterone, such as hormone replacement therapy, birth control pills, and even hormones for early pregnancy support, they often say they feel drowsy.

True, not every woman reports fatigue or nausea. The ones that do may just be more sensitive to their hormones. Some describe fatigue out of proportion to how pregnant they are, to the point where they can't get out of bed. For-

Buy a humidifier. It adds moisture to the air, which is helpful for coughs.

Rest. Go to bed early. Sleep in. Nap. Call in sick. "Trying to keep on working when you're sick is working against your body," Dr. Burns says. If you return to the office too soon, you may have a relapse.

Drink. You need lots of fluids when your body is fighting off a virus. Colds are often accompanied by fever, which increases your breathing rate and makes you sweat more. Additionally, your body is trying to get rid of the waste products created in the battle between your immune system and the infection. All of this can lead to dehydration, says Dr. Burns. To stay hydrated, drink enough hot tea, water, and juices to make you go to the bathroom every 2 hours on average.

Choose C. When you have an infection, take 500 to 1,000 milligrams of immune-boosting vitamin C hourly up to six times daily. If you experience diarrhea, slowly cut back to an amount that you can tolerate, says Dr. Suther-

tunately, often the women who suffer the most describe the most dramatic improvement when the first trimester ends.

Many women survive those 3 months by being good to themselves. They stay in bed later and go to bed earlier. They do low-impact exercise. They modify their work environment—but even that can be stressful if they haven't shared the news with their employer or coworkers. The stress often subsides around the time women start feeling better physically and decide it's okay to share their pregnancy with people.

Expert consulted: Shari Brasner, M.D., obstetrician-gynecologist in private practice, New York City, and author of *Advice from a Pregnant Obstetrician*

land. Vitamin C has been shown by many studies to reduce the duration of cold and flu symptoms.

Try echinacea. Take a dropperful of this immune-enhancing herb in tincture form (more effective than the pill form) hourly at the first sign of a cold or flu, suggests Liz Sutherland, N.D., a naturopathic physician with the National College of Naturopathic Medicine's Natural Health Sciences Research Clinic in Lake Oswego, Oregon. Chase the herbal extract with a glass of juice if the taste bothers you.

See a doctor. If your mucus is green or yellow, you may have a sinus infection and may require antibiotics.

The Effects of Fibromyalgia

After a Saturday spent raking leaves, hauling mulch, and hiking up and down a soccer field, only a superwoman with arms of steel wouldn't be tired and sore, right?

Don't be so quick to explain your pains away.

For some, muscle soreness and fatigue may signify something more serious than weekend overexertion. It could be fibromyalgia, a chronic disorder that results in muscle pain, sleep problems, and fatigue.

"Fibromyalgia feels like the worst case of flu ever imaginable," says Carole Kenner, D.N.S. (doctor of nursing science), professor, and director of the Center for International Affairs at the University of Cincinnati, who has fibromyalgia herself. Other symptoms include morning stiffness, regular headaches, bowel problems, jaw pain, and chemical sensitivities to smells such as perfume or cigarette smoke.

One result—or symptom—of fibromyalgia is that you may not have enough serotonin, a neurotransmitter that regulates your sleep and perception of pain. Women with fibromyalgia also may have low levels of cortisol, a hormone that gives us the energy for "flight or fight." But there is plenty of a chemical known as Substance P, which may intensify pain perception.

Complex and still not fully understood, fibromyalgia is easy for doctors and patients to miss. "The sleep problems and fatigue make it easier to dismiss as everyday aches and pains," says Dr. Kenner. "We think, 'I must have picked up my child wrong' or 'I must have carried something too heavy.'"

We sometimes blame our fatigue on a bad night's sleep—a common complaint among fibromyalgia patients, who often have trouble either falling or staying asleep.

In many ways, fibromyalgia resembles chronic fatigue syndrome, leaving some to speculate the two conditions are simply different points on a spectrum. Like CFS, fibromyalgia affects primarily women, has an unidentified cause, and has symptoms that include pain, fatigue, sleep problems, and cognitive difficulties.

Also like CFS, fibromyalgia is a diagnosis of exclusion: Your doctor must rule out all other causes for your fatigue and pain. She'll also do a "tender point" exam, checking the sensitivity of 18 specific areas on your body. If you've been in chronic pain for at least 3 months and have tenderness in 11 or more areas located near your knees, elbows, buttocks, and the base of your skull, you've probably got fibromyalgia.

Some doctors suspect fibromyalgia is "triggered" by an infection, injury, or stress that somehow affects the central nervous system. Others blame an out-of-whack immune system in perpetual overdrive.

Many women with fibromyalgia have symptoms for 5 to 7 years before they're diagnosed. If you don't want to spend the next decade feeling inexplicably exhausted, start looking for a doctor who's knowledgeable about fibromyalgia. The Fibromyalgia Network (www.FMNetNews.com or 800-853-2929) maintains a list of fibromyalgia-friendly health care providers. You might also want to try the rheumatology department at a nearby medical school.

Once you find a doctor, talk to her about therapies—both conventional and alternative—as well as lifestyle modifications that can help. Commonly used medications include antidepressants—which may reduce your pain and help you sleep as well as boost your mood—since depression often accompanies fibromyalgia. Although nonsteroidal anti-inflammatory drugs (NSAIDs) are often prescribed to ease the muscle pain of fibromyalgia, there's no proof that they work, and they may even make you feel worse by leading to intestinal problems that result in food allergies, an overactive immune system, or even irritable bowel syndrome.

Alternative practitioners, such as naturopaths and chiropractors, take a slightly different approach to fibromyalgia. Instead of focusing on the symptoms, they try to correct the underlying nutritional or physiological problems that may be causing the disease. Their recommendations may include the following:

SAM-e (S-adenosyl-L-methionine). More commonly used for treating osteoarthritis, SAM-e (found in health food stores) can also act as an antidepressant and a pain reliever for fibromyalgia patients. Doses up to 1,200 milligrams daily are considered safe. This supplement may increase blood levels of homocysteine, a significant risk factor for cardiovascular disease. To keep homocysteine levels down, take SAM-e with folic acid and vitamins B_6 and B_{12}.

5-HTP (5-Hydroxytryptophan). Besides reducing the number of painful "tender points," this nutritional supplement may help with the pain, stiffness, and fatigue of fibromyalgia by providing the precursor for the serotonin you lack, says Dr. Sutherland. The typical dosage is 300 to 900 milligrams per day, usually divided into two or three doses. Some research suggests that taking 100 milligrams of 5-HTP three times a day, as well as St. John's wort extract (300 milligrams standardized to 0.3 percent hypericine three times a day) and magnesium (200 to 250 milligrams three times a day), produces very good results, according to Dr. Sutherland. The form of magnesium is very important, she adds. "I recommend magnesium citrate, malate, succinate, or fumarate."

Make sure you purchase a reputable brand of 5-HTP. In the past, some brands of this supplement were found to contain trace amounts of a contaminant that caused serious symptoms associated with eosinophilic myalgia syndrome (EMS). The following brands were confirmed to be free of the contaminant: Natrol, Nature's Way, TriMedica, Country Life, and Solaray.

Chiropractic. In one small study, 15 to 30 sessions of chiropractic manipulation eased pain, reduced fatigue, and improved sleep in a group of women with fibromyalgia.

Food Sensitivities: A Hidden Energy Sapper

Food allergies (more accurately known as food sensitivities or intolerances) can sap your energy just as much as ragweed season does.

"When you have a sensitivity to a food, your body doesn't break it down fully," says Liz Sutherland, N.D., a naturopathic physician with the National College of Naturopathic Medicine's Natural Health Sciences Research Clinic in Lake Oswego, Oregon. As a result, these incompletely digested food molecules sneak into the bloodstream. Your body then treats them as foreign invaders and fires up the same defenses it would for a cold virus.

"This constant low-grade immune response is very irritating," Dr. Sutherland says. You feel tired and foggy—because all your energy is going toward fighting off that ice cream cone you ate this afternoon.

If you suspect you have a food sensitivity, cut the questionable food out of your diet for 4 to 6 weeks. (Common offenders are dairy, soy, corn, and gluten, which is found in wheat, oats, rye, barley, couscous, and other grains.) Then slowly reintroduce the food and see how you feel. If you eliminate more than one item, allow 3 days between adding each food back into your diet.

You can also ask your doctor to test you for food sensitivities, but if you tend to have a delayed allergic reaction to certain foods, you may be out of luck—some food allergy blood tests pick up only on immediate immune responses.

Acupuncture. This ancient Chinese practice, which involves inserting needles at specific points in the body, may temporarily relieve the pain and morning stiffness of fibromyalgia. The National Institutes of Health, after reviewing numerous studies, concluded that acupuncture "may be useful as an adjunct treatment" for fibromyalgia.

As with CFS, there are several things you can do that may improve your condition, including exercise, relaxation techniques, and cognitive behavioral therapy. In one study, researchers found nondrug therapies such as CBT and exercise provided more energy and pain relief in fibromyalgia patients than did antidepressants, muscle relaxants, or NSAIDs.

When Lupus Is to Blame

No two women are alike—especially when it comes to an autoimmune disease like lupus. In fact, three women with lupus can talk and discover they have no symptoms in common.

With lupus, the immune system attacks the body's own tissues and cells, causing swelling and pain. In some women, it's constant. Others have cycles of remission, where they feel healthy and well, and relapses, when the disease "flares." Some women experience severe fatigue. Others may start losing their hair. If you have lupus (shorthand for systemic lupus erythematosus), you may experience these symptoms as well:

- Joint and muscle pain
- Unexplained fever
- Skin rash on the face
- Chest pain when breathing deeply
- Fingers and toes that turn colors when you're cold or stressed

- Unusual sensitivity to the sun, with 15 minutes of exposure resulting in sunburn, fatigue, or joint pain
- Swelling in the legs or eyes
- Swollen glands
- Recurrent and frequently multiple canker sores.

"If you have at least three of these, it's probably worth seeing a doctor," says Rosalind Ramsey-Goldman, M.D., associate professor of medicine at Northwestern University Medical School in Chicago.

Whatever your symptoms, you are sure to feel worn out from your body's fight against itself. The inflammation may be one reason for the fatigue, but the sleep problems or the anemia that often goes along with a chronic disease like lupus could be to blame.

Lupus's prevalence among women, and especially women between ages 15 and 45, has many experts suspecting hormones as a player, particularly estrogen. Lupus also seems to have a slight genetic link, so if you have a family history of lupus, let your doctor know.

Other theories blame stress, sunlight, drugs, and viruses for the disease.

As tough as lupus is for researchers to understand, it's often just as hard for family members, who are often unwilling to pick up the slack for a mom who doesn't look or sound sick to them. You don't get sympathy the way someone with crutches and a cast might.

You may have to see more than one doctor to get the help you need. While rheumatologists specialize in diseases such as lupus, you may need a nephrologist for kidney problems or a dermatologist for rashes. Among prescription treatment options are the following:

Steroids. Fast and effective, steroids are usually the first line of therapy for serious lupus flares. But they may increase your risk of osteoporosis, diabetes, high blood pressure, and other conditions, so many doctors look for other options.

Immunosuppressive drugs. Medications such as Rheumatrex or Imuran may be easier on your body than steroids alone, says Dr. Ramsey-Goldman. "Sometimes two drugs at lower doses give you better control with fewer side effects." But if you choose this route, you should discuss with your doctor vaccinations against tetanus, hepatitis B, and the flu. That's because these "steroid-sparing drugs" treat lupus by suppressing your overactive immune system. Your lupus will be under control, but you'll be at greater risk for colds, the flu, and anything else that comes around.

Antimalarials. Used for treating malaria, drugs such as Plaquenil also help the skin and joint problems associated with lupus by reducing inflammation and ratcheting down your hyperactive immune system.

NSAIDs. Nonsteroidal anti-inflammatory drugs such as Motrin, Advil, and Aleve can ease the pain, swelling, and fever of lupus. But talk to your doctor before buying a bottle of over-the-counter ibuprofen; you may need a higher dosage than the one listed on the label.

Other strategies include the following:

Stay in the shade. Sunshine can trigger a flare. To protect yourself, stay inside from 10 A.M. to 2 P.M., when the sun's rays are the strongest. Other times, wear a hat, long sleeves, and an SPF-30 sunscreen.

Take notes. Cognitive problems with memory or concentration represent a common challenge for women with lupus. Keep your edge by carrying a small notebook and a pen to jot down everything from your grocery list to phone numbers.

Exercise. "You need to get regular rest, but that doesn't mean the rest of the time you're a lump," says Joan Merrill, M.D., chief of rheumatology at St. Luke's–Roosevelt Hospital Center in New York City. She urges women to pursue moderate exercise such as walking, swimming, and bicycling. "When people have a chronic illness and let themselves waste away, they only get sicker."

Be heart smart. Lupus patients may have an increased risk of heart disease, making it especially important that they eat a heart-healthy diet low in saturated fat, control their blood pressure, and watch their cholesterol.

Find good fatty acids. Research has shown that omega-3 fatty acids, found in fish such as sardines and salmon, and gamma-linolenic acid (GLA, present in black currant oil and primrose oil) can reduce the painful inflammation of autoimmune diseases such as rheumatoid arthritis and lupus. Researchers are uncertain how the fatty acids work, but one theory about evening primrose oil is that it blocks the effects of prostaglandins, body chemicals that cause inflammation.

Mark Stengler, N.D., director of natural medicine at Personal Physicians clinic in La Jolla, California, and associate clinical professor at the National College of Naturopathic Medicine in Portland, Oregon, recommends at least 3 grams of omega-3 fatty acids and 150 to 400 milligrams of GLA daily for those with inflammatory conditions like lupus and arthritis. Check how much GLA your evening primrose oil contains to determine the exact dosage. He also suggests taking both of these fatty acids at the same time—particularly if you plan to keep taking them for more than a few months; naturopaths believe that long-term solo use may create an essential fatty imbalance in the body, which could worsen existing conditions.

Drink your milk. Both the steroids used to treat lupus and the physical inactivity too commonly associated with it can increase your chances of osteoporosis. Take 1,200 to 1,500 milligrams of calcium a day split into two doses, says Dr. Ramsey-Goldman, because your body can absorb only so much calcium at one time. She also suggests increasing your intake of dairy products like low-fat cheese and yogurt.

Energy and Emotions

It's a Monday, and Carolyn drags herself out of bed, feeling oddly numb (in addition to exhausted). She goes through the motions of getting the kids off to school and herself to work, but the feeling remains. It scares her—for it reminds her of that bad spell she had 2 years ago, that blanket of despair that seemed to suffocate her.

It started right around the time her mother began demanding more time and energy. Her daily routine, already insane, grew worse, with regular calls and visits to ensure her mother's needs were met. Added to the pressures of work and of raising two children, the extra duties sent her over the edge.

Months passed, and she found it harder and harder to get out of bed. She no longer looked forward to going to work, and there were days she'd sit in her car and cry. When she got home in the evening, she felt like she had nothing left for her husband or children. All she wanted to do was sleep. Yet most nights she'd lie awake for hours. If she did fall asleep, her eyes would snap open at 4 A.M., and that would be the end of rest for the night. Eventually, her husband convinced her to see a doctor.

After 6 months of medication and talk therapy, Carolyn felt better and stopped treatment. Now, 2 years later, she's wondering if her old nemesis—depression—is back.

Carolyn is right in viewing her sleep problems and fatigue as possible warning signs of depression, says Laura J. Miller, M.D., chief of the Women's Services Division at the University of Illinois at Chicago.

Nearly everyone who is depressed—and many who suffer from other mental disorders—has disturbed sleep patterns of some sort, she says. It may be difficulty falling asleep, sleeping too much, nightmares, middle-of-the-night awakening, or other irregular sleep patterns.

"It's an individual thing, so everybody needs to do a personal appraisal," says Catherine A. Chambliss, Ph.D., psychology professor and department chair at Ursinus College in Collegeville, Pennsylvania. "But I urge people to take disrupted sleep somewhat seriously, to recognize that a good night's sleep will have an effect not only on your energy the next day but also on your cognitive and emotional functioning."

Fatigue or Depression?

If you're merely worn-out from juggling responsibilities and running all over the place, you generally going to sleep pretty well and wake up feeling refreshed and energized after a good night's sleep, says Dr. Chambliss. Like many overscheduled women, you might have a little difficulty going to sleep, but your body will try its best to restore itself.

"Women who aren't depressed and who are busy with their careers and their families realize that their lives have tremendous meaning," says Dr. Chambliss. "They recognize the value of what they're doing and, if they're lucky, are appreciated by others for what they're doing."

On the other hand, "the hallmarks of depression are hopelessness and helplessness," she says. "It's chronic despair and the inability to do anything about it. If you start finding yourself feeling that there's nothing you can do but give up, it's usually time to see a physician or therapist."

The symptoms of clinical depression, according to the National Mental Health Association, are the following:

- A persistent sad, anxious, or "empty" mood
- Sleeping too little or sleeping too much
- Reduced appetite and weight loss or increased appetite and weight gain
- Loss of interest or pleasure in activities once enjoyed
- Restlessness or irritability
- Persistent physical symptoms that don't respond to treatment, such as headaches, chronic pain, or constipation and other digestive disorders
- Difficulty concentrating, remembering, and making decisions
- Fatigue or loss of energy
- Feeling guilty, hopeless, or worthless
- Thoughts of death or suicide.

If five or more of these symptoms last longer than 2 weeks or if the symptoms are severe enough to interfere with your daily routine, you should see a doctor.

Depression: A Woman's Nemesis

When we're depressed, our brains are affected in two ways. First, the neural circuits in our brains that are responsible for sleep, moods, thinking, appetite, and behavior fail to function properly. Second, critical neurotransmitters—the chemical messengers that enable brain cells to communicate with one another—fall out of balance.

The effects of depression on sleep can be measured on an electroencephalogram (EEG), which consistently shows a delayed rapid eye movement (REM) cycle among depressed patients. When we're deprived of REM sleep—the dream state—we become far more emotional, reactive, and unstable.

Patients with other mental disorders also don't function as well when they're not sleeping well, says Dr. Chambliss. "One of the functions of sleep is to stabilize emotional reactivity, and if sleep is being disrupted by mental disorders, there can be measurable consequences," she says.

Another reason for sleep problems is that when we're depressed, we spend more time sitting and fretting, and so we don't tire our bodies out for a good night's sleep. We may respond to our fatigue in a passive way, such as consuming more alcohol or caffeine and smoking a lot. Paradoxically, some depressed people sleep more than usual because sleep becomes a means of escape, says Dr. Chambliss. Whatever the symptoms, it's clear our reactions are working against our body's rhythms.

All in the Hormones?

Over the course of a lifetime, about 1 in 5 women will be diagnosed with depression, compared with only 1 in 10 men.

Why the difference? One reason may be our hormones. One study by the National Institute of Mental Health showed that the depressive mood swings of premenstrual syndrome resulted from an abnormal response to normal hormone changes during the menstrual cycle. Women with a history of PMS experienced relief from their depressed moods when their sex hormones, estrogen and progesterone, were temporarily "turned off" by a drug that suppresses the function of the ovaries.

The symptoms returned within a week or two after the hormones were reintroduced. Women with no history of PMS had no effects from the hormonal manipulation, which indicates that sex hormones don't cause PMS—they trigger PMS symptoms only in women with a vulnerability to the disorder. Researchers still are trying to determine what makes some women suffer from PMS and not others.

Additionally, many women who are depressed have an overactive hormonal system that regulates their body's response to stress. Normally, when we're threatened physically or psychologically, the hypothalamus—the brain region that manages hormone release from our glands—increases production of corticotropin releasing factor (CRF). That stimulates the pituitary and adrenal glands to release more of their hormones, thus preparing our body for "fight or flight."

Our bodies respond with reduced appetite, decreased sex drive, and heightened alertness. This is a good reaction in the face of real danger, but research suggests that persistent overactivation of this hormonal system may leave us exhausted and lay the groundwork for depression.

Low levels of serotonin and norepinephrine also seem to play an important role in mental disorders. Women naturally have lower serotonin levels than men, which may be one reason we're more prone to depression. That may also partly explain the sleep disorders of depression. Higher levels of serotonin increase the amount of deep sleep we get every night and improve our overall well-being. When levels drop—as they do when we're depressed—sleep is disrupted.

Types of Depression

Depressive disorders can take many forms, but there are three common types.

Major depression. Women with this form of depression often have a combination of symptoms that interfere with work, study, sleep, eating, and the ability to enjoy once pleasurable activities. These depressive symptoms last for at least 2 weeks, and they can trigger recurring thoughts about suicide or death. An episode may occur only once, but often it recurs. If you have symptoms like these, see your doctor immediately.

Dysthymia. A milder but more lasting depression, dysthymia can go untreated for years, draining happiness and energy from our lives and the lives of those around us. Symptoms may be the same as for a major depression but often are long-term and may just make others think we're grouchy or gloomy. We may be constantly pessimistic, guilt-ridden, irritable, withdrawn, or easily hurt by others, for no apparent reason. We may have trouble getting along at home, work, or school. Professionals don't usually assume a woman has dysthymia until she's been depressed for most of the day, more days than not, for at least 2 years—a long time to be miserable.

Bipolar disorder. Also called manic-depressive illness, it is characterized by mood swings between highs and lows. Sometimes the mood switches are dramatic and rapid, but most often they are gradual. In the depressed cycle, you can have any or all of the symptoms of depression. In the manic cycle, you may be overactive, overtalkative, and filled with energy, often misguided.

Why You're Tired in Winter

The holidays completely wipe us out. We eat more, drink more, and socialize more, which makes us tired. And we tend to exercise less.

Sometimes, just the feeling of being trapped inside makes us depressed, especially in areas where the winters are severe. We want to stay in bed and pull the blanket over our heads until spring arrives. In the Northeast and the Midwest, social activities are curbed. People don't plan things because the weather is so unpredictable.

For some, the problem may be seasonal affective disorder (SAD), in which a lack of sunlight causes depression. SAD most often begins in late fall or early winter and goes away by summer. It occurs more often in northern climates, and it's four times more common in women.

Symptoms of SAD may be similar to those in other forms of general depression—increased appetite, especially a craving for sweet or starchy foods; weight gain; a

An inability to sleep, sometimes for days, or a decreased need for sleep is one of the symptoms in the manic phase. Other symptoms include inappropriate displays of excitement, high energy level, the need to talk constantly and loudly, racing thoughts, distraction, sudden increase in sexual desire, impaired judgment, embarrassing behavior, and dangerous risk taking.

Know Thyself

If you've had one type of mental disorder at some time in your life, you're more likely to experience another, so it's important to keep a finger on the pulse of your mental health. In fact, after one episode of depression, there's a 50

heavy feeling in the arms or legs; a drop in energy level; fatigue; a tendency to oversleep; difficulty concentrating; irritability; and avoidance of social situations. If the winter blahs seem to be affecting your daily life, it's time to see a doctor.

Your doctor may suggest light therapy, in which you sit under or near a specially made light box or a light visor for 30 minutes each morning. She may also recommend medication or behavior therapy, either by itself or with light therapy.

One way to help prevent SAD in winter is to get sun on your face by going for a midday walk outside, says Alice D. Domar, Ph.D., a Harvard Medical School psychologist and director of the Mind/Body Center for Women's Health at the Mind/Body Institute in Boston.

Whatever the cause, continue to exercise. It will make you feel better, reduce depression, and make you healthier.

percent chance of a recurrence; after two episodes, that risk increases to 75 percent.

Equally important is to not let sleep disturbances and fatigue go unnoticed—or to try to drown out problems with alcohol or other drugs.

"When a lot of people hit problems in life, they use alcohol to help them relax and fall asleep," Dr. Chambliss says. Although alcohol may help you fall asleep, it also can wake you up in the middle of the night and make falling back to sleep difficult. Thus, alcohol deprives you of your full sleep cycle, which can result in emotional problems.

Drinking alcohol can become a vicious cycle. You drink because you're stressed, then you don't sleep well and you're tired the next day. So you drink more to relax and get to sleep, thus leading to a stream of poor sleeping nights and increasing the risk, or severity, of depression or anxiety disorder—a panic attack that can leave your heart pounding, your breathing labored, and you feeling faint and dizzy. Both depression and anxiety disorder can become more serious when coupled with increased alcohol consumption.

Similarly, you may consume more caffeine because you're tired—and that, too, can disrupt sleep patterns, Dr. Chambliss says. You should also be aware that as you age, you may not handle caffeine or alcohol in the same way you did when you were younger.

Seek Solutions

If you're concerned that you may be depressed, start with a visit to the doctor to rule out any medical conditions or medications that may cause symptoms similar to depression. Some—including anemia, thyroid disease, and calcium imbalance—are common among middle-aged women. Even women who have adjusted their diets to eat more iron can suffer from anemia during perimenopause because the blood loss during prolonged, heavy periods is greater than they're accustomed to, Dr. Miller says.

If your physical health is fine, the next step is a psychological evaluation from a psychiatrist or a psychologist. Research shows that most of the 19 million Americans who suffer from a depressive illness each year can be helped if they get appropriate treatment.

You can go the alternative route or the traditional route or combine the two.

Traditional therapies include the following:

Short-term therapy. Typically involving 10 to 20 weekly sessions, this is best used when your symptoms are mild but have been around for a while and are causing consistent unhappiness. It is also used with anxiety disorders to teach you to change specific actions and change your thinking patterns.

One of the two main types, cognitive behavioral therapy focuses on changing negative styles of thinking and behaving. Instead of thinking everything is going to go wrong on a given day, you begin to think of yourself as worthy and look for the good in your life.

Interpersonal therapy focuses on problems in your personal and social relationships. The therapist helps you see how you interact with other people and works on changing that behavior to improve relationships. For example, if you feel like your husband and children walk all over you, you'll learn how to express your needs and get them met.

Long-term psychodynamic therapies. Best used with severe depression, these therapies attempt to resolve internal conflicts. You look inside yourself to uncover and understand emotional conflicts. That may involve looking back at unresolved problems from childhood, such as abuse or neglect, and trying to work them out. It may last for months or years, as long as you and your therapist think you are improving and growing as a result of the therapy.

Most patients with moderate to severe depression do best with a combination of medication to relieve symptoms quickly and psychotherapy to learn more effective ways of dealing with problems. Commonly used medications include the following:

Antidepressants. You probably know someone on Prozac—it's practically the birth control pill of the new millennium in terms of its pervasive use. The first in a new generation of antidepressants, it has been nearly as life changing for those suffering from depression as the Pill was for women who didn't want to get pregnant.

Prozac is the brand name for fluoxetine, one in a class of drugs called selective serotonin reuptake inhibitors (SSRIs), which also includes Paxil, Luvox, and Zoloft. These and other newer medications that affect neurotransmitters like dopamine, serotonin, and norepinephrine generally have fewer side effects than tricyclics, the older class of depression drugs. To find the right drug for you, your doctor may have to try several medications or dosages. Also note that it could take as long as 8 weeks on the medication before you feel the full therapeutic effect.

Lithium. For years, lithium was the drug of choice for treating bipolar disorder. It was scary stuff because the

Medications That Affect Your Sleep

Psychotropics—medications that affect your mental state—usually have one of three effects on sleep:

- They make it easier to sleep, by treating an underlying condition.
- They are sedating.
- They make it more difficult to sleep.

The most commonly used psychotropics are antidepressants, which are also prescribed for anxiety disorders and eating disorders. Tricyclics are the oldest antidepressants still in use and tend to be sedating. When they're effective, your sleep patterns improve even before you begin to feel better, says Laura J. Miller, M.D., chief of the Women's Services Division at the University of Illinois at Chicago.

Tricyclics may, however, make you feel groggy during the day. They also might not be a good choice if you are already exhausted from pregnancy or parenting small children or if you're sleeping too much because of depression.

range between an effective dose and a toxic one is narrow. Now, however, several other drugs have been found to control mood swings, and anticonvulsants such as divalproex sodium (Depakote) and carbamazepine (Tegretol) are generally considered the first choice for treating acute mania. Both can have serious side effects, such as lowered white blood cell count, skin rashes, gastrointestinal disturbances, and liver dysfunction, so careful monitoring is necessary.

Benzodiazepines. Although antidepressants are also used to treat some anxiety disorders, such as panic attacks and phobias, more commonly used is this class of drugs,

The most widely prescribed antidepressants are selective serotonin reuptake inhibitors (SSRIs), such as Prozac. Although they eventually help you reclaim normal sleep patterns, they can initially make sleep more difficult. They can make you nervous and jittery for 2 to 3 weeks, and some women need sleeping pills to get them through that adjustment period, says Dr. Miller.

Newer antidepressants, such as Effexor, affect other neurotransmitters in the brain. Because they're more balanced, their effects on sleep are more unpredictable. They can be sedating or activating or have no effect on sleep.

Communicate with your doctor about any problems you're having with medications, including troublesome sleep changes. Be as detailed as possible. Keep a sleep journal, or ask your doctor for a mood chart, on which you track your mood, sleep, and medications.

which includes alprazolam (Xanax), diazepam (Valium), and chlordiazepoxide (Librium, Librax, Libritabs). These antianxiety medications help to calm and relax you while clearing troubling symptoms. Benzodiazepines are generally prescribed for brief times—days, weeks, or intermittently—because you can become dependent on them and have withdrawal reactions when you stop taking them.

Buspirone (BuSpar). This is another antianxiety medication sometimes prescribed for general anxiety. It must be taken daily for 2 or 3 weeks before its effects are felt. For specific reasons, other medications may occasionally be prescribed for anxiety disorders, including antihistamines, barbiturates such as phenobarbital, and beta-blockers such as propranolol (Inderal, Inderide).

Alternative Treatments

There are nondrug treatments, such as the following, that can also help your problems.

Get out and exercise. Any kind of exercise is good, but getting outside is best, because nature and sunlight have a way of lifting spirits.

Exercise can complement traditional treatments in those who are clinically depressed and prevent depression in those who don't have the illness. One study of hospitalized depressed patients found significant reductions in depression among patients who participated in an aerobic exercise program, but not in a control group who did only occupational therapy. Another study found improvement in a group of patients assigned to 8 weeks of walking and jogging, with no improvement in those assigned to recreational therapy or a waiting list.

Any form of exercise may work, though most studies have been conducted with running, walking, or other aerobic exercise. One study found similar improvements between groups who ran and those who lifted weights for 8 weeks. That study also concluded that mood improvement did not depend on achieving physical fitness.

How exercise eases depression remains unclear. Psychologically, exercise may give us a greater sense of mastery, important when we feel loss of control over our lives, says Dr. Miller. An analysis of 51 studies linked exercise to a small but significant increase in self-esteem. It also gets our minds off what's bothering us. And it may improve our health, physique, flexibility, and weight, which puts us in a better mood, she adds. Just being able to eat more without worrying about gaining weight can increase our pleasure and sense of self-control.

Intense exercise has been shown in some studies to increase brain serotonin. And beta-endorphins, chemicals that reduce pain and can make us euphoric, have been linked to the "runner's high" that comes after intense exercise (we're talking serious sweat here).

One thing's clear: Exercise, completed at least 4 to 6 hours before bedtime, makes us sleep better. A controlled clinical trial of 32 depressed adults found that a program of weight-training exercise three times a week for 10 weeks improved the quality of participants' sleep and lessened their depression.

Socialize. Walking with a friend or a group is doubly beneficial, because you get the exercise and the bonus of conversation and company. People who aren't willing or likely to depend on others and people who are hostile or aggressive, and who thereby have fewer friends and social support systems, are more apt to relapse into major depression, according to a University of Washington study.

"Social support is a tremendous buffer against depression," says Alice D. Domar, Ph.D., a Harvard psychologist and director of the Mind/Body Medical Institute in Boston. "And with today's working moms, time with her friends is the first thing to go." We also tend to isolate ourselves when we're depressed. So reach out. Attend classes, concerts, lectures, church or synagogue, book clubs, or anything else that suits your personality.

Get religion. One recent study conducted by Patricia Murphy, Ph.D., assistant professor in the department of religion, health, and human values at Rush–Presbyterian–St. Luke's Medical Center in Chicago, shows that having religious beliefs lowers levels of depression and has an even greater mitigating effect on hopelessness.

Relax. Numerous studies have shown that meditation, guided imagery, and muscle relaxation alleviate symptoms of anxiety and depression. Dr. Miller suggests that one way to relax is with a quick abdominal exhalation of breath—one or two every second. Relax on the inhale. Breathing with the abdomen and diaphragm calms the sympathetic nervous system, which regulates our blood pressure and pulse, making us feel more relaxed and energized, Dr. Miller says. A therapist trained in these areas can tailor a regimen of exercise and relaxation to suit your particular disorders and symptoms, she adds.

Turn to herbal therapy. Hypericum, the concentrated extract from St. John's wort (*hypericum perforatum*), is used in Germany more than any other medication to treat depression. German researchers say it is safer than the antidepressant drug imipramine and just as effective for treating moderate depression, with fewer side effects.

Although St. John's wort is sold as a dietary supplement at health food stores in this country, the Food and Drug Administration does not allow any antidepressant claims. The National Institutes of Health, however, is conducting a 3-year study on its effectiveness and proper dosages.

Try Chinese medicine. It combines the use of herbs and acupuncture and may help with depression and anxiety. "A practitioner would put together a treatment plan that may include a course of acupuncture treatments and an herbal formula tailored to address your specific experience of depression," says Rosa Schnyer, Lc.Ac., a licensed acupuncturist in Tucson, Arizona, and a research specialist in the University of Arizona's psychology department.

Chinese medicine focuses not on treatment of specific diseases but on trying to balance the "life force," or "Chi," says Schnyer. And it doesn't try to separate psychological from physiological symptoms. So it wouldn't be necessary for a licensed acupuncturist to attribute your lethargy directly to depression, anxiety, or fatigue. Rather, the acupuncturist would try to understand how your personal experience of fatigue, combined with other symptoms, affects your life and would design a treatment to correct this imbalance.

The acupuncturist would select certain points along the surface of your body and insert small, fine needles to supplement what is empty and drained and to correct obstruction and blockage from the areas where the energy is stagnant. In addition, she might create an herbal prescription and make dietary and lifestyle recommendations.

Even with treatment—whether through medication, psychotherapy, or alternative treatments—it can take months to recover from depression or anxiety disorders. You can expect your mood to improve gradually; in the meantime, nurture yourself and let family and friends help you.

"It's a shame to let depression go untreated," says Dr. Chambliss. "The majority of people who seek help show dramatic improvement in a relatively short time."

PART THREE

Energy Chargers

Sleep: The Holy Grail

It's 5 P.M., and Carolyn is anxious to leave work. If she can make it home early, she just might get to bed at 9 instead of midnight. Suddenly, her boss pops into her office, needing help with some memos for a meeting later tonight.

Her stomach churns. "I was here late last night. And the night before," Carolyn mutters as she grudgingly plops her bags on the floor and restarts her computer. "When will I ever get any rest?" she asks herself.

Bleary-eyed and exhausted, she plods through the assignment and finally drags herself home at 7:30 P.M.

All she can think of is crawling into bed and getting some sleep.

But first she has to eat, review her son's homework, clean the kitchen, and call her mom. By the time she dots the last "i" and crosses the last "t" on Michael's book report, it's nearly midnight. Desperate to get some shut-eye, Carolyn pops a sleeping pill and calls it a night.

Sleep Defined

Sleep experts recommend that we get at least 8 hours of sleep each night. Yet the average woman age 30 to 60 sleeps only 6 hours and 41 minutes a night during the workweek. No wonder we fantasize about a good night's sleep more often than a dip in the hot tub with Harrison Ford.

Like food, clothing, and shelter, sleep is a basic human need that we can't live without. It's considered an altered state of consciousness that restores us physically and emotionally. And it is as essential to our long-term health as daily exercise, says Kathy Sexton-Radek, Ph.D., a sleep medicine specialist and professor and chair of the psychology department at Elmhurst College in Illinois.

Researchers aren't sure how or why sleep renews us, but they do have some ideas. Sleep lowers body temperature, decreases oxygen consumption, and slows heart rate and metabolism (the rate at which we burn calories) 5 to 25 percent. It may be that these changes force our bodies to conserve energy overnight so that we feel rejuvenated in the morning, says Suzanne Woodward, Ph.D., an expert on women and sleep and assistant professor of psychiatry at Wayne State University School of Medicine in Detroit.

Another theory is that sleep gives our brains a much-needed rest from the flurry of daily activity, says Margaret Moline, Ph.D., director of the Sleep–Wake Disorders Center at New York Presbyterian Hospital in New York City. It's like a Zamboni for our brains, clearing away the detritus of the day even as the giant machine clears the pitted ice. If our brains didn't have the opportunity to sleep, we wouldn't be able to concentrate or think so clearly, says Dr. Moline.

Sleep is vital to learning, too. In a study of 27 people that looked at one night's sleep, researchers found that those who got enough of the right kind of sleep had an easier time learning and retaining information than did those who didn't. Researchers defined "the right kind" as about 8 hours of sleep that included deep, slow-wave sleep in the first 2 hours of slumber and at least 2 hours of deep REM sleep in the early morning.

Sleep is also important for emotional balance. When we get enough restful sleep, we're less likely to snap at our husbands, yell at our kids, or kick the pet. We're also less sluggish. In fact, missing as little as 2 hours of sleep every night for a week makes our levels of fatigue, confusion, and anxiety skyrocket and causes mood swings, according to researchers from the University of Pennsylvania School of Medicine. The reason is that sleep loss causes daytime sleepiness, which makes us struggle to stay awake, alert, and motivated to do anything that requires energy. And that has a negative effect on our mental health.

When you think of the perfect good night's sleep, you might imagine fluffy pillows, a cozy blanket or comforter, sweet dreams—and no alarm clock to startle you into wakefulness in the morning. But there's a lot more to catching some zzzs than you might think.

Soon after you crawl into bed, you begin a complex but fascinating journey that takes you through four stages and two distinct types of sleep: REM (rapid eye movement) and non-REM.

Usually occurring about five times during the night, REM sleep is that part of the sleep cycle where we dream, subconsciously fantasizing about winning the lottery and buying that mansion in Maui. Our brain waves hit warp speed, as if we were awake. Our eyes bounce back and forth like Ping-Pong balls, and we actually get a mini-cardiovascular workout as our hearts beat faster and we breathe harder. "It's like stepping on the accelerator while your car engine is running to give it more gas," says Dr. Sexton-Radek. But even though our brains and bodies are "active" during REM sleep, it is still restful sleep. And everyone experiences it—even those who swear they don't dream.

We spend about 25 percent of the night in REM sleep. The rest is non-REM sleep, which occurs in four stages.

Demons in the Night

If you're snoozing 8 hours and still don't feel rested, you may have a sleep disorder like one of the following. See your doctor right away.

Sleep apnea is the second most common sleep disorder after insomnia. Obstructive sleep apnea occurs when the throat muscles and tongue relax so much during sleep that partial blockage of the airway occurs. You can actually stop breathing 5 to 100 times an hour. Central sleep apnea occurs when your brain fails to send certain signals to your diaphragm and chest muscles to initiate breathing. As a result, you wake up several times a night to catch your breath. Mixed apnea is a combination of the two.

The most effective treatment is continuous positive airway pressure (CPAP). You wear a mask over your nose that's connected to a machine that pumps pressurized air in to keep your airway open during sleep. Several dental devices that prevent your tongue from sliding backward are also available. Surgery may also be used to increase the size of your airway, but the procedure is only 30 to 50 percent effective.

Narcolepsy is a chronic neurological disorder whose signs include overwhelming daytime sleepiness, sleep at-

Each stage of the non-REM part of the cycle is necessary to help replenish physical and mental energy, sharpen memory and the ability to learn, and restore us emotionally. If we skip a stage or fail to remain in any particular one long enough, we wake up bone-tired and cranky. Yet all stages work in sync to help refresh and energize us.

Stage 1. We enter this phase of non-REM sleep when we first fall asleep. A light doze, it's a transition between

tacks with or without warning, brief episodes of muscle weakness or paralysis triggered by strong emotional reactions, and frightening dreamlike images that occur while falling asleep or upon awakening. Depending on the symptoms, treatment includes drugs that stimulate the central nervous system and antidepressants.

Restless legs syndrome causes creepy, crawly, tingly feelings in your legs that often compel you to walk, stretch, give yourself a massage, or perform knee bends for relief. Daytime sleepiness, fatigue, and difficulty falling asleep or staying asleep are also common.

Mild symptoms are usually relieved by regular exercise, massage, hot baths, heating pads, or ice packs or by eliminating caffeine. Moderate to severe cases call for prescription medications.

Nocturnal sleep-related eating disorder compels you to gorge on large quantities of food late at night while half-asleep or wide-awake. It's most prevalent among obese women who are under stress and who may have other sleep disorders. Treatment involves prescription drugs like dopamine agents, benzodiazepines, and antidepressants.

wakefulness and sleep during which our muscles relax. Brain wave activity is similar to when we're awake, because we're not really asleep. It lasts a mere 1 to 7 minutes and starts the cascade of sleep.

Stage 2. During this stage, a slightly deeper sleep, brain wave activity and body mechanisms begin to slow. This is what sleep experts actually call "sleep." Again, we're in this stage for 1 to 7 minutes.

Stages 3 and 4. Although they are defined as separate stages, sleep experts still lump these two stages together because the differences between them are so slight. It is during these deeper stages—known as delta, or deep, sleep because of their association with slow brain-wave patterns—that our immune systems are at their best, reacting with a surge of energy to produce white blood cells that fend off bacteria and viruses. "That's why if you get enough rest during a cold or the flu, you're more apt to

The Ideal Mattress

Restful sleep depends on a comfortable bed. To find a mattress that's right for you, test-drive a few at a bedding store. Spend at least 20 minutes lying on your back, your side, and your stomach to determine whether the mattress offers great support or is too hard or too soft, says Mary Ann Keenan, M.D., director of neuro-orthopedics in the department of orthopedic surgery at Albert Einstein Medical Center in Philadelphia. Choices to consider:

Firm mattress. If you experience occasional back pain or have arthritis, a firm coil mattress with a soft surface is the way to go, says Pamela Adams, D.C., a chiropractor and yoga instructor at Magnolia Chiropractic in Larkspur, California. You get great back support, and the soft surface cushions your hips, knees, and shoulders. If you can't find one with a soft surface, place a 2-inch-thick piece of foam over the mattress and add a mattress pad, Dr. Adams suggests.

Stay away from soft mattresses. They're bad for your back and neck, and they make it difficult for you to get out of bed without straining your arms and shoulders, says Dr. Keenan.

fight the infection," says Dr. Sexton-Radek. Along with REM sleep, these two stages are the most restorative because this is when our bodies turn on the switch for many of our necessary functions, including the release of hormones and neurotransmitters.

When we first fall asleep, we go through non-REM stages 1 and 2 and then have our first REM. After that, we go through non-REM stages 1 through 4 and then have our second REM. The entire pattern is repeated throughout

Foam mattress. This can support your back just as well as firm coil bedding. A mattress with a 34-pound compression ratio (a measure of firmness) may do the trick, but always let your back decide. For a firmer feel, try a mattress with a higher ratio. The drawback is that over time the pressure and heat of your body may cause changes in the foam that affect the mattress's ability to give you the support you need, says Dr. Keenan.

Waterbed. It conforms to your exact shape and gives your body customized support. But if you have arthritis, a waterbed can be difficult to get into and out of, especially in the morning, when joints are sore and stiff, says Dr. Keenan. A waterbed is also not good if you have a problem with motion sickness.

Air mattress. It's good as long as it's filled with enough air to make it firm. An air mattress works well for those who are prone to bedsores and other skin irritations because they can't turn themselves over in bed. Although the mattress is firm, the surface is soft enough to prevent abrasions on the skin, says Dr. Keenan.

the night. In all, we typically have five REM episodes, which usually last 4 to 12 minutes each but can last up to 30 minutes.

The 10 Commandments of Sleep

There are things we do (or don't do) that affect how quickly we fall asleep and how well we sleep. Following these 10 Commandments of Sleep will lead to blissful rest, energized mornings, and sweet dreams.

1. Thou shalt not drink alcohol or caffeinated beverages within 4 to 6 hours of bedtime. A nightcap before bed may help you conk out faster, but it can shorten the time you spend in the deeper stages of sleep and cause you to wake up several times during the night. It can also cause nightmares and early-morning headaches. One reason for the middle-of-the-night awakening is that your nervous system becomes aroused as your blood alcohol level drops.

As for caffeine, it stimulates the brain. So don't be surprised if you find yourself staring at the ceiling in the wee hours if you had an after-dinner cup of coffee. Cola, chocolate, cocoa, and certain prescription drugs also contain caffeine. Moderate daytime use usually doesn't interfere with sleep, but if you have trouble falling asleep or staying asleep, cut it out completely, Dr. Woodward says. While most people's systems clear the caffeine from a cup of coffee in 3 to 5 hours, others need as many as 10 hours.

2. Thou shalt not smoke cigarettes within 4 to 6 hours of bedtime. Like caffeine, nicotine stimulates the central nervous system. It interferes with falling asleep and staying asleep by increasing heart rate, blood pressure, and adrenaline levels, says Amy Wolfson, Ph.D., cochair of Women in Sleep and Rhythms Research (WISSR) at the College of the Holy Cross in Worcester, Massachusetts.

3. Thou shalt not nap for longer than 30 minutes. The urge for that midafternoon snooze is associated with your body's internal biological clock. Between 2 and 4 P.M., a drop in body temperature occurs, which usually causes you to feel sleepy, says Terri E. Weaver, R.N., Ph.D., associate professor at the University of Pennsylvania School of Nursing and a sleep researcher at the Center for Sleep and Respiratory Neurobiology at the University of Pennsylvania School of Medicine, both in Philadelphia. A 20- to 30-minute nap works wonders if you didn't get enough shut-eye the night before.

One Swedish study found that eight participants who were deprived of sleep and then allowed to take a 30-minute midafternoon nap the next day reported feeling more alert. They performed better on tests than when they weren't permitted to take a nap. As seen in this study, naps can help make up for lost sleep. "If you slept for 7 hours last night but need 8 hours to feel your best, a half-hour nap can help put you back on track," says Dr. Moline. "But it won't make up for a 5-hour sleep deficit accrued the prior week."

Just stick with an afternoon nap. Snoozing too late in the day will make you less sleepy at your normal bedtime. And don't doze more than 30 minutes. If you nap longer than that, you'll fall into the deeper stages of sleep and feel even groggier when you wake up. Choose a room for your nap that is dark and quiet. If you nap regularly, always do it at the same time, Dr. Moline says. Just be aware that those who nap on a regular basis often sleep less at night and then can become sleep-deprived if they start missing their naps, she adds.

4. Thou shalt not exercise within 3 hours of bedtime. As you wind down in the evening, your body temperature falls to get you ready for sleep. Aerobic exercise and weight training do just the opposite. They raise your temperature, boost your heart rate, speed your breathing, and increase levels of the stimulating hormone adrenaline. This prevents you from falling asleep at your normal bedtime, says Dr. Weaver.

It's best to exercise in the morning because that helps you sleep better at night, says Dr. Weaver. Researchers don't know why, but they suspect that expending a burst of energy early in the day tires out the body just enough so that sleep comes more easily at night.

5. Thou shalt not sleep in on weekends. Changing your sleep patterns on the weekends resets your internal clock. "Hitting the sack late on Friday and Saturday night, and then sleeping in on Saturday and Sunday, will prevent you from getting to sleep at your normal bedtime. So you'll wake up tired on Monday morning," says Dr. Weaver. Plus, it won't make up for the 5- to 8-hour sleep deficit you may have accumulated the week before. The corollary to this commandment: Thou shalt go to bed at the same time every night and get up at the same time each day.

6. Thou shalt not lie awake in bed for more than 15 minutes. If you can't fall asleep, chances are you'll watch the clock, toss and turn, and become anxious. This will make falling asleep that much more difficult, says Dr. Woodward. The better alternative is to get up, leave your bedroom, and do something relaxing like reading or watching television. Keep the lights dim and the noise down, and make sure that whatever you read or watch doesn't excite you. Return to bed only when you feel drowsy.

7. Thou shalt not bathe less than 2 hours before bedtime. Whether you take a cool shower or soak in a hot bath, you can alter your body temperature. Remember that a natural dip in temperature helps cue your body that it's time to sleep. "Bathing too close to bedtime may throw off that natural cue," Dr. Woodward says.

Do You Wake Up with a Headache?

Most morning headaches are triggered by daytime tension or stress. Even though you're relaxed while you sleep, those 7 to 8 hours aren't enough to undo the chronic tension some of us experience during the day.

Fatigue is another factor. One study found that those who endured ongoing tension and migraine headaches were more tired than those who didn't. Part of the reason was that those with headaches didn't sleep as well. They took longer to doze off and woke up more often during the night.

Chronic headaches can interfere with falling asleep and staying asleep. And the fatigue you experience the next day often makes the pain even worse, creating a vicious cycle.

There's also a link between morning headaches and high blood pressure. Overnight decreases in blood pressure result in the dilation of arteries in your head. As your heart works overtime to pump blood throughout your body, your brain gets an added dose that it doesn't need, resulting in pulsating head pain.

Another possibility is sleep apnea, a common sleep disorder characterized by loud snoring and brief interruptions in breathing while sleeping. The lack of oxygen and changes in blood pressure that result cause the headache.

Experts consulted: Kathy Sexton-Radek, Ph.D., sleep medicine specialist and professor and psychology department chair, Elmhurst College, Illinois, and Suzanne Woodward, Ph.D., expert on women and sleep and assistant professor of psychiatry, Wayne State University School of Medicine, Detroit

8. Thou shalt not use your bed for anything other than sleep or sex. Reading, watching television, or doing office work in your bedroom can leave you feeling alert and make it more difficult to fall asleep, which is not the best emotional state to be in when you finally turn out the lights. "You want to associate your bedroom with tranquillity and calm, not with tension or entertainment. Reading the last chapter of a murder mystery or becoming aggravated at the evening news may keep you awake," says Dr. Moline.

9. Thou shalt design thy bedroom for rest. Flip through any department store catalog and you're bound to find the picture-perfect bedroom that you wish you had in your own home. Notice that there are no computers, fax machines, or televisions crowding the view. And everything matches. You can create the same environment.

First, ditch the hardware, software, and boob tube. Consider purchasing a color-coordinated bed ensemble that includes a comforter, dust ruffle, pillow shams, and matching sheets. The matching linens help calm the setting for sleep. Buy draperies to match, and make sure they have blackout linings to keep the room as dark as possible when it's time to sleep, says Charlotte Thompson, president and owner of Charlotte Thompson and Associates, an interior design company in Dallas. Look for shades and drapes with blackout linings at any window treatment retailer that offers custom drapes.

Select calm, soothing colors from the blue and green families. Reds, oranges, and yellows tend to stimulate rather than relax you, says Thompson. Opt for incandescent or halogen lighting instead of fluorescent. Halogen is closer to natural light, which is softer on the eyes.

Consider aromatherapy. Use relaxing, soothing scents like lavender, bergamot, chamomile, vanilla, and sandalwood in your bedroom. Place 1 drop of essential oil on a handkerchief and sniff, or dab it on your sheets. Put 5 drops in some bathwater and soak. Or put 4 drops in a pan of hot water and inhale before you go to bed. If you experience skin irritation, discontinue using the oil.

10. Thou shalt dress appropriately for bed. Wear whatever is comfortable for you: a silk negligee, a flannel nightgown, a cotton T-shirt. Or sleep in the buff. But keep in mind that your body temperature drops prior to falling asleep, rises during the night, then falls before you awake. So always think lighter rather than heavier when choosing pajamas. If you have perimenopausal symptoms such as hot flashes and night sweats, wear cotton pajamas, Dr. Woodward suggests.

Food: The All-Day Energizer

It's another Monday morning, and Carolyn is up at 6 A.M. As usual, she feels groggy, light-headed, and weak. Her brain is working about as well as a cotton-stuffed piccolo.

Still bleary-eyed even after her shower, she stubs her toe on a barstool in the kitchen. Aggravation adds to fatigue as she pours the kids' cereal and orange juice in between feeding the dog and loading the dishes from last night's late-night ice cream fest into the dishwasher.

There's no time for a real breakfast of her own, so she brews a pot of coffee strong enough to etch diamonds, pours it into her travel mug, and grabs a chocolate-covered doughnut for the road.

By the time she gets to the office, the caffeine and sugar have kicked in and she's got enough energy to get through the first three items on her to-do list. But by the time the staff meeting starts at 10, she's dragging again, so she joins her coworkers at the office coffee pot for another cup of brew and a slice of the crumb cake someone brought from home.

Lunch is a fast-food bacon cheeseburger, fries, and soft drink devoured in the car as she hits the dry cleaner, video store, and library. By 2 P.M., however, she can barely keep her eyes open. So she grabs another cup of coffee and a candy bar.

As soon as the clock strikes 5, Carolyn hits the door. With sports practice tonight for both kids and a stop by her mom's, plus the fact that Ben is out of town again, dinner tonight will be late (after 7 P.M.)—and takeout.

It's a classic catch-22 situation: We're too tired to eat right, but unless we eat right, we won't have the energy we need, and if we don't have the energy we need, we won't eat right.

"If you're not eating a nourishing diet, you're just not going to run at your optimal level," says Phyllis Woodson, R.D., C.D.E., a registered dietitian at the Strelitz Diabetes Institute and in the division of maternal-fetal medicine at Eastern Virginia Medical School in Norfolk. Woodson counsels women about their eating habits. Many of her clients, she says, complain of fatigue. There's no surprise there, when you consider the following:

- Up to 39 percent of premenopausal women have low iron levels. While a full-blown deficiency, or anemia, causes fatigue and general weakness, research suggests that even levels not low enough to be classified as anemia may impair performance.
- Nearly half of all women in the United States get less than the recommended Daily Value of vitamin B_6, a B-complex vitamin responsible in part for peak mental and physical performance.
- In one study of 350 healthy women conducted at Arizona State University in Tempe, researchers found that 30 percent had low blood levels of vitamin C, another key fatigue-fighting vitamin.
- Are we hungry—or tired? With our nonstop lifestyles, says Baltimore dietitian Colleen Pierre, R.D., it's easy to mistake one for the other.

"We're rushed," Woodson says. "We're at the computer, we're in our cars, we're on our car phones." When it comes to what we're eating, she says, a lot of women "are just sort of winging it."

In the process, they're shortchanging themselves on the energy-enhancing qualities of eating right. Like the wood that feeds a fire, the calories in food fuel every part of our bodies, from our brains to our muscles. For peak energy, we have to use high-quality fuel. That means a balance of vegetables, fruits, whole grains and pastas, lean meats, low-fat dairy, and small amounts of fats. And research suggests that how we combine those foods may be just as important for energy as the foods themselves. Even the size or timing of meals may affect concentration, energy levels, and sleep.

Eat Already

Before we even begin with what and when we're eating, however, we need to make sure we *are* eating.

"I see it a lot," says Pierre, who has interviewed women around the country about their eating habits. "Women go all day without eating. Or they eat as little as they can."

Not eating starves our brains, which makes concentration difficult, writes Pamela Smith, R.D., in her book *The Energy Edge*. That's because to function properly, the brain needs the energy that comes from glucose, which comes from food. That fuzziness often translates into fatigue.

So we come home at night, ravenous and weary, and binge on whatever is convenient: cookies, cakes, pepperoni pizzas. Worried about the pounds that come with this out-of-control nighttime eating, we continue to avoid food during the day.

And as for getting a balanced diet, with enough fruits, vegetables, whole grains, fiber, vitamins, and minerals . . .

fahggedaboudit! Only about 17 percent of us eat the recommended five or more fruits and vegetables a day.

Repeated nutritional skimping, whether for months or even years, leaves us chronically tired, irritable, headachy, or moody and sets us up for serious illnesses ranging from diabetes to heart disease to cancer. It's akin to putting inferior fuel in our cars. As every good mother would say: Eat already!

But not too much. Because the heavier we are, the more energy we require just to move—in fact, to function every day. Basically, being overweight is a physical burden.

"Carrying extra weight is a drag," says Pierre. Think about hauling a couple of 20-pound dumbbells up three flights of stairs. Imagine how exhausting it would be to carry them around all day. That's about how it feels to weigh an extra 40 pounds.

One study of more than 40,000 women showed that gaining a mere 5 to 10 pounds may bust our energy supplies. In a questionnaire, weight gainers said they were less able to perform routine daily tasks, such as vacuuming, than women who lost similar amounts of weight.

Being overweight can drain us even while we sleep. Our lungs are forced to work harder, and fatty tissue in our throats can keep us from getting plentiful doses of energizing oxygen.

So the keys are those two bastions of nutritional health: balance and moderation.

Basic Beginnings

The best place to begin eating right is with breakfast. Unfortunately, only one in four of us is starting there, says Elizabeth Somer, R.D., in her book *Food and Mood: The Complete Guide to Eating Well and Feeling Your Best.* And of those who *are* eating breakfast, one-third eat this most important meal of the day away from home—and often in the car.

"The grab-and-go approach has made it even tougher to find a healthy breakfast," notes a report by the Center for Science in the Public Interest (CSPI), a nonprofit

Coffee: Energy Sapper in a Mug

If you're feeling a little run-down, the culprit may be your cup of coffee. Although this caffeine-spiked beverage can give you a morning jolt and chase the fuzzies from your brain, it can also send you crashing later in the day.

Caffeine's stimulating effects kick in within 30 minutes, leaving you more energetic. But later, you feel sluggish and muddleheaded as your body reacts to mild caffeine withdrawal. Caffeine is also a diuretic, causing dehydration, which can make you feel fatigued.

Caffeine inhibits the absorption of vitamins and minerals like iron and calcium, which are important for energy. And it can interfere with sleep, leaving you drained the next day, says Nancy Fishback, M.D., associate professor of medicine at the Sleep Disorders Center at Eastern Virginia Medical School and Sentara Norfolk Hospital in Virginia.

It's best to limit caffeine from coffee, tea, chocolate, and other products to 300 milligrams a day, Dr. Fishback says. That's one to three 5-ounce cups of your run-of-the-mill coffee. (Coffee-bar brews can pack as much as 550 milligrams in one serving.) Be aware that some prescription and over-the-counter drugs also contain caffeine.

Cut your caffeine habit slowly. Giving it up abruptly is likely to cause headaches. One suggestion: Mix half decaf coffee and half regular. Or try "light" coffees, which contain less caffeine.

group that explores nutritional issues. "Most takeout breakfasts are nutritional nightmares."

CSPI likely would call that doughnut Carolyn grabbed as she ran out the door "dessert for breakfast," since its prime ingredients (sugar and fat) do nothing for long-term energy. Instead, it's likely to drag her down.

With that little palm-sized piece of fried cake, Carolyn is getting one-fourth of her entire day's quotient of fat, one-fifth of all the calories she needs, and unhealthily large dollops of artery-clogging saturated fat and cholesterol. What she's *not* getting is a balanced mix of stick-to-her-ribs fiber, cell-building protein, and all-important vitamins and minerals.

If only she had reached for the bran cereal. In one British study, eating cereal in the morning put volunteers in a better mood, enabled them to perform better on a spatial-memory test, and resulted in their feeling calmer at the end of the tests than those who hadn't eaten cereal. Another study showed less fatigue in people who ate a low-fat, high-carbohydrate breakfast (like high-fiber cereal with fat-free milk) than in those who ate any other combination of fat and carbohydrates.

Sugar as Energy Snatcher

Carolyn's doughnut is also loaded with 7.9 grams of sugar, which sets her up for that nutritional crash-and-burn at 10 A.M. Forget the myth about sugar's boosting energy. Although sugar (also known as glucose) does initially boost blood sugar levels (and therefore makes more energy available to cells), the effects disappear quicker than a week's pay at an amusement park.

Sugar releases all of its energy at once into the bloodstream, causing your blood sugar level to soar. This results in a spike of the hormone insulin, which then pushes the sugar into blood cells. The glucose is immediately absorbed and just as quickly disappears, and the blood sugar level drops, often ending up lower than it was before you ate the doughnut or candy bar. The dizziness, headache, and fatigue that follow are from low blood sugar.

In one study at Kansas State University of 120 women, researchers gave some participants 12 ounces of water and gave others drinks sweetened with either aspartame or sugar. Within 30 minutes, those who had drunk the sugar-sweetened brew were sleepiest.

Sugary foods contain few nutrients. So if we fill up on sugar, we crowd out the vitamins, minerals, antioxidants, and other food components that help us feel and look good. No wonder Carolyn's reaching for the crumb cake at 10 A.M.

If she'd munched a low-fat whole wheat bran muffin with a banana, however, she'd probably have been fine until lunch. Complex carbohydrates like that muffin are burned more slowly, so there's no quick blood sugar spike or resulting crash. They keep us going and going, like little battery-powered bunnies.

Fatiguing Fat

That doughnut also contains a significant amount of fat, and most of it is the truly bad for your heart trans fats, which are created when hydrogen is whipped into liquid vegetable oils to make them solid. They're extremely unhealthy; studies show that trans fats significantly increase the risk of developing coronary heart disease.

Plus, too much fat slows you down and robs you of energy by creating a kind of sludge in your bloodstream, says Smith. Your body is so busy digesting and storing excess fat that it actually slows blood circulation, reducing the delivery of oxygen to your cells.

You don't want to avoid fat entirely, however. Not only do you need it to transport vitamins and produce hormones, but at 9 calories per gram (compared with 4 per gram for carbohydrates and protein), fat packs slowly digested energy that gives your meals staying power.

Carolyn should also have had more protein at breakfast, such as a glass of low-fat milk or a cup of yogurt. Protein helps stabilize energy levels by working with carbohydrates and fats to regulate blood sugar, says Smith.

"There's a symphony effect with all of them being there together that moderates blood sugar," says Linda Barnes, M.S., R.D., a registered dietitian in Virginia Beach, Virginia.

You can make a simple but healthy breakfast in 5 minutes, Somer says in her book. Even a slice of vegetable pizza served with a large glass of orange juice fuels you through the morning as well as a bowl of cereal would.

In fact, vitamin C—found in oranges, cantaloupe, and other fruits and juices—is a proven energy booster. When you're short on this critical vitamin, fatigue is one of first symptoms to appear. One reason may be that vitamin C helps your body absorb iron, a mineral that carries energizing oxygen to your cells. One 8-ounce glass of orange juice more than meets your daily requirements for C.

For a balanced, energy-boosting start to your day, the CSPI offers these suggestions.

- Stuff half a whole wheat pita with ½ cup low-fat cottage cheese and sliced peaches, pears, or bananas.
- Roll up a tortilla with scrambled eggs and salsa. (For a quick scrambled egg, coat a microwave-safe bowl with cooking spray, lightly beat 1 egg and 1 tablespoon milk, and microwave on high for 90 seconds.)

- Melt a thin slice of low-fat cheese over a sliced tomato on a whole wheat English muffin.
- Stir ½ cup each of plain low-fat yogurt and orange-pineapple-banana juice with ⅓ cup sliced bananas and a handful of fresh or frozen blueberries. Freeze overnight.
- Combine ¼ cup low-fat ricotta with ½ cup applesauce and a dash of cinnamon. Sprinkle with Grape-Nuts.

Water Is Nature's Energizer

"To maintain energy, you need water," says Barbara Gollman, R.D., a nutrition consultant in Dallas and spokesperson for the American Dietetic Association. But don't wait until thirst strikes to drink up. By then your water levels are depleted enough to drag you down. One small study of bicyclists showed that performance dropped when they lost as little as 2 percent of their weight in fluids.

The standard recommendation: Drink at least 8 cups a day—more if it's hot out or if you exercise, take certain medications such as diuretics for high blood pressure, are ill, or drink alcohol or caffeinated beverages like coffee, says Linda Barnes, R.D., a registered dietitian in Virginia Beach, Virginia.

Milk, juices, soups, fruits, and vegetables also contain fluid. And while most decaffeinated beverages replenish fluids, caffeine and alcohol drain your water stores. (If you must drink them, quaff an extra cup of water for each cup of coffee or glass of wine.)

You know you're getting enough liquids if your urine is straw-colored, not bright yellow.

Maintain Balance at Lunch

Regardless of how healthy breakfast was, your blood sugar and energy levels still begin to lag about 4 hours later.

Time for lunch.

There's really nothing wrong with the fast-food burger Carolyn gulped for lunch—but from now on she should order it sans heavy sauces, double cheese, bacon, and fries and add a salad or a couple pieces of fruit and substitute low-fat milk for the sugary soft drink.

Lunch carries with it its own smoking gun: the afternoon slump. To a certain extent, we're going to feel a bit drowsy in the early afternoon regardless of what we eat—that's just due to our circadian rhythms. But what we eat can worsen their effects.

This is where balance comes in. If you chow down on something like fettuccine Alfredo, chances are you'll be drooling all over your expense reports by 2 P.M.

That's because you've just eaten a meal composed almost entirely of carbohydrates and fat. Carbohydrates aren't all bad. In fact, they're the best source of energy and are found in everything from candy bars and soft drinks to beans, fruit, and vegetables. It's only when you eat too many carbs, have the wrong kinds, or eat them alone, without a bit of protein, that you gain weight or feel sluggish.

Additionally, eating more than about 1,000 calories at any one meal forces your body to work harder just to digest them. There's a *reason* everyone retires to the comfort of the living room for a post-dinner snooze on Thanksgiving.

Also, every time you munch something like a bagel, a big plate of pasta—or that huge holiday feast of turkey, mashed potatoes, stuffing, and gravy—your brain produces a neurotransmitter called serotonin, which has a calming effect. If you eat too much of a serotonin-boosting food, however, you'll watch that calmness morph into catatonia.

But add a bit of protein to smaller meals—say, by substituting clam sauce for the cream sauce on that pasta—and you can curtail serotonin's sleepy-time effects. That's because most proteins (meat, dairy, beans, fish) boost our brain's supplies of dopamine and norepinephrine, neurotransmitters shown to enhance alertness. One British study showed that protein actually moderated the effects carbohydrates had on serotonin.

That's why most experts suggest combining small amounts of protein, fat, and carbohydrate at meals—hence the need for balance.

In fact, in one study of 18 volunteers, those who ate a lunch of cheese sandwiches and milk shakes in which the carb, protein, and fat intake was balanced were less drowsy, uncertain, and muddled (and more cheerful) than those who ate lunches tipping the scales in terms of fat or carbohydrates.

So a hamburger on a bun meets the basic balance requirements—a good mix of protein (the burger), carbohydrate (the bun), and not too much fat.

But there are major players missing: fruits and vegetables.

Not only do they provide a plethora of vital minerals and vitamins, but they also contain hundreds of phytonutrients—substances such as lycopene, lutein, carotenoids, and indoles—that appear to have tremendous effect on not only energy but overall health.

Yet women don't even come close to getting enough fruits and vegetables. On average, we eat about 3.6 servings a day—perhaps one apple, ½ cup of string beans, and a glass of orange juice—well below the nine most nutritionists recommend we eat. And no, french fries don't count.

Think yellow, orange, dark green, and leafy.

"Vegetables are the Cadillac of your food," Woodson

says. "If you're not tapping into vegetables, it's to your detriment."

Ideal lunches include the following:

- A small bowl of canned low-fat minestrone soup and 2 ounces of turkey on whole wheat bread with lettuce and mustard, served with 8 ounces of skim milk.
- A tossed salad with ¼ cup canned kidney beans, 1 ounce low-fat cheese, and 3 tablespoons low-fat dressing, with 2 slices sourdough bread and a glass of sparkling water.
- A peanut butter crunch sandwich (2 tablespoons peanut butter mixed with 1 tablespoon wheat germ and 2 teaspoons honey, spread on multigrain bread) served with 8 ounces of skim milk and 1 cup of fresh strawberries.
- Three ounces of extra-lean roast beef on a whole wheat roll with tomato, lettuce, and mustard. Add 1 piece of fruit and 1 cup of raw cauliflower florets, sliced carrots, and broccoli florets.

Snack Success

One way to banish fatigue and mental fogginess is to eat mini meals every 2 to 3 hours throughout the day.

In a study conducted at Tufts University in Boston, healthy, older women (average age 72) ate meals of 250, 500, and 1,000 calories. Their blood sugar levels rose and then rapidly returned to normal—as desired for sustained energy—only after the 250-calorie snack.

But we're not talking candy bar, cookies, or chips for that midafternoon snack. Snacks should follow the same guidelines as the rest of your meals: a mix of protein, carbohydrates, and fat, with minimal amounts of fats and processed sugars.

Individualized Energy Programs

Here are special circumstances that make eating for energy a challenge—and ways to cope with them.

I need to feed my family, and we don't like the same foods. Don't just microwave a variety of frozen dinners—many are packed with sodium and fat and fall short on vegetables, says Jayne Hurley, R.D., senior nutritionist at the Center for Science in the Public Interest in Washington, D.C. A better idea: frozen meal kits in a bag. Many are lower in fat and sodium, easy to fix, and taste terrific. And they have a decent amount of energy-boosting vegetables, so you get vitamins A and C, fiber, and more.

I eat out frequently. A study by researchers at the University of Memphis and Vanderbilt University showed that women who ate out more than five times a week consumed more energy-sapping calories, sodium, and fat than women who ate at home.

When possible, says Hurley, order from "light" menus. Go for grilled, baked, or blackened, instead of fried. Choose sandwich wraps enclosing fresh vegetables; nix the cheese unless you opt for the low-fat variety. And beware of salad dressings. The typical chef or Caesar salad with

And watch the calories in snacks. "We've lost sight of portion size," says Jayne Hurley, R.D., senior nutritionist at CSPI. Our cookies, cakes, and beverages are bigger than ever. "I call them 'sweets on steroids.'"

In one CSPI sampling, a popular cookie purchased at a shopping mall contained 750 calories and 48 grams of energy-stealing fat.

So think about how much food you normally eat during the day and divide it into smaller portions, says Barnes. If

dressing contains more than half the fat you need in an entire day.

I'm very overweight. Being overweight is an energy drain, says Linda Barnes, R.D., a registered dietitian in Virginia Beach, Virginia. Add to that a tendency to forgo nutrient-dense fruits, vegetables, and grains in favor of cakes, cookies, and fried foods—or hardly any food at all—and there's little fuel to keep you going.

Give yourself a jump start by combining light exercise—a walk around the block, perhaps—with balanced meals containing fewer calories. Draw an imaginary line down the plate, says Colleen Pierre, R.D., a registered dietitian in Baltimore. Fill half the plate with vegetables. Put nutrient-dense starches like brown rice or whole-grain pasta on one quarter of the plate, and lean meat, chicken, or fish on the remaining quarter.

Also keep a food diary for a few days, Barnes suggests. Use a pocket-size calorie book to add up the daily tallies. Giving up just 200 calories a day—a pat of butter and a half glass of wine—can let you drop a pound a week. This slow, steady weight loss keeps you from feeling calorie- and energy-deprived, Barnes says.

you brought yogurt, a tuna sandwich, and an apple for lunch, save the yogurt for a 3 P.M. snack.

Eat for Sleep

Given the late dining hour in Spain, it's amazing Spaniards get any sleep at all. What we eat soon before bedtime can come back to haunt us worse than a bad job performance.

There are the obvious culprits, such as caffeine and alcohol, both of which can disrupt the quality and duration of sleep. But even chocolate and peppermint can mean a 2 A.M. wake-up call. Eaten within 2 hours before you go to sleep, they can cause gastric reflux in the night, says Nancy Fishback, M.D., of the Sleep Disorders Center at Eastern Virginia Medical School and Sentara Norfolk Hospital in Norfolk, Virginia. Your stomach acid churns and rises, splashing into the top of your esophagus or throat, waking you up with a burning, upset stomach or a chronic cough.

Forget the cake, ice cream, and other rich foods or big meals before bedtime, too, Dr. Fishback says. Because rich, sugary foods wreak havoc with blood sugar levels well into the night, they also disrupt sleep. All those carbs raise blood sugar, remember. In comes insulin to flush out the sugar. When its level falls, you may feel hungry again—enough to wake you up and send you stumbling to the fridge.

So Carolyn's likely to become reacquainted with that greasy fried chicken dinner or chocolate mousse cheesecake at some point in the night.

If you must eat within 2 hours of bedtime, try an ounce of low-fat cheese, a cup of low-fat yogurt, or a hard-boiled egg. Add a half-dozen whole wheat crackers or a piece of fruit and a small handful of macadamia nuts or some avocado.

Sometimes, however, there's just no avoiding that late-night meal. In that case:

- Wait an extra hour or so before bedtime to give your body a chance to digest your food. That way, you're less likely to worsen that nasty gastric reflux.
- Raise the head of your bed so you sleep propped up a bit. This may keep those gastric acids from waking you in the night.

Carolyn Revisited

Carolyn realizes her diet is out of whack and visits a nutritionist. Two months later she's sleeping better and has more energy during the day, and she's even dropped a couple of pounds.

Here is a sampling of the energy-revving nutritional plan Carolyn has adopted.

Breakfast: 1 slice of whole wheat bread, 1 ounce of low-fat cheese and an apple.

Midmorning: 5 whole-grain crackers and 1 cup of nonfat strawberry yogurt.

Lunch: 1 pear, 1 baked potato with 1 teaspoon of butter, 2 or 3 ounces of grilled chicken, 2 cups of fresh raw spinach topped with raw carrot slices, broccoli, mushrooms, and nonfat salad dressing.

Midafternoon: ½ cup of plain yogurt mixed with 1 tablespoon of raspberry all-fruit spread.

Late afternoon: ½ cup of trail mix that Carolyn makes at home and stores in a sealed plastic bag. The mix: 1 cup unsalted dry-roasted peanuts, 1 cup unsalted dry-roasted shelled sunflower seeds, and 2 cups raisins.

Dinner: 1 cup of vegetable soup, 1 cup of cooked cauliflower, ½ cup of brown rice, 3 ounces of lean fish sautéed in 1 teaspoon of canola oil, and 1 cup of raw carrot sticks.

A couple of hours before bedtime: ¾ cup of toasted oats cereal and ½ cup of skim milk.

Herbs: Energy
the Natural Way

The bright yellow poster fairly screams its message at Carolyn: Feeling Tired? Boost Your Energy TODAY the Natural Way! Intrigued, she wanders over to the display of herbal bottles and boxes, all sporting nearly unpronounceable names, all promising to banish fatigue, energize her, do just about everything except turn her hair blond.

She picks up one of the bottles. Whoa! Pricey. Twenty dollars for a month's supply of leaves? Then she thinks about how she's been feeling lately and, figuring she's worth it, heads to the checkout counter.

Hold on there, Carolyn. That bottle of herbal remedies may seem like a lifesaver right now, but it's "false energy," says Marie Mulligan, M.D., a clinical researcher at Santa Rosa Kaiser Permanente in California. Stimulating herbs like ephedra (also known as *ma huang*), yerba maté, and guarana that are touted as a quick energy fix have very little long-term effect on energy, she says.

"Americans have this misplaced idea that having energy is just about being able to keep going. What you're doing is acquiring an energy debt. If you're going to take ephedra, you may as well save your money and have a cup of coffee, because either way it's just a temporary stimulating effect," Dr. Mulligan says. These remedies can also dehydrate you, which *contributes* to fatigue. And you shouldn't take ephedra if have high blood pressure, glaucoma, heart problems, diabetes, or thyroid disease.

Using Herbs

The first thing you need to do, says Ellen Kamhi, R.N., Ph.D., a professional member of the American Herbalists Guild and coauthor of *The Natural Medicine Chest*, is figure out how you like to use herbs.

You can cultivate your own. Teaching yourself about herbs and how to prepare infusions, decoctions, and tinctures can be therapeutic in itself. "But never use a plant from the wild that you have not positively identified," says Dr. Kamhi.

If it's convenience you're after, capsules and tinctures are the way to go. A well-stocked health food store is likely to have everything you need. Before buying a packaged herb product, check the ingredients. High-quality preparations have very few additives. Things like pharmaceutical glaze, titanium dioxide, and yellow dye number 5 have no place in an herbal preparation, says Dr. Kamhi. "In general, the better brands are usually more expensive," she says.

If you're buying loose herbs, you can tell if they're fresh and of high quality by taking a good sniff. The natural aroma of the herb should come through loud and clear. And whenever possible, says Dr. Kamhi, choose organic herbs.

Overall, about 27 percent of Americans use complementary therapies, including herbs, to treat fatigue, and about 26 percent use herbs to treat insomnia, according to a study in the journal *Sleep Medicine Reviews*.

Instead of trying to jolt your body into action, Dr. Mulligan and other herbalists suggest turning to herbs that will support overall well-being, encourage relaxation, and gently nurture you back to a refreshed state. Here's their top 10 list.

Nettle (*Urtica dioica*)

Though you might think of nettle as just an annoying plant with a powerful sting, this ancient herb is also a marvelous tonic. Herbal tonics work gently and slowly to improve overall health. Some improve and support general health and well-being and help you overcome periodic stresses and illnesses, while others act upon specific systems of the body to improve overall functioning.

Historically, nettle has proved its mettle as a fiber for making cloth and rope. During World War I, German soldiers' overalls often were made of nettle fiber. And from a culinary standpoint, nettle has been used for centuries— added to soups, eaten as a vegetable, even made into a beer. Containing calcium, vitamins A and K, and chlorophyll, it's also an excellent source of iron. Though scientific research has focused on nettle's potential for treating prostate disease and tuberculosis, herbalists prize nettle as a general tonic, particularly for women.

Herbalist Aviva Romm, a certified professional midwife, executive director of the American Herbalists Guild (AHG), and author of *The Natural Pregnancy Book*, recommends nettle to all women: young, old, pregnant, and menopausal. "Within 20 minutes of drinking nettle tea, they feel energized," she says, "and it's not like the temporary boost of chocolate or coffee. It's sustained energy." Nettle balances and regulates blood sugar, she says, so with regular use—at least 1 cup daily to get the benefit and up to 2 cups a day—it helps to prevent blood sugar crashes and sugar cravings. Nettle also provides significant amounts of minerals, and clinical evidence suggests that it nourishes the adrenal glands, which sit atop the kidneys and produce adrenaline all day in moderate amounts. That's what gets you up in the morning and keeps you going throughout the day.

How to use it. You can eat nettle as a vegetable, Romm says. Simply steam or sauté lightly and add butter, garlic, lemon, or tamari (a form of soy sauce). She also suggests making an infusion by putting 4 tablespoons of dried nettle leaves (organic is best) in a quart jar filled with near-boiling water. Steep for an hour and then strain. If the spinachy taste doesn't appeal to you, add some miso, tamari, or even a bouillon cube. You can also use the infusion as a broth base for soup or stew. The plants are available at some herb specialty shops and by mail order.

Ginseng (*Panax ginseng, Panax quinque- folius,* and *Eleutherococcus senticosus*)

Ginseng actually refers to several different roots. In descending order of intensity, there are Asian (*P. ginseng*), American (*P. quinquefolius*), and Siberian (*E. senticosus*) ginseng. Ginseng is one of a group of herbs known as adaptogens—tonics that have a general beneficial effect on the body.

For women, Ellen Kamhi, R.N., Ph.D., a professional member of the AHG in Oyster Bay, New York, and co-author of *The Natural Medicine Chest*, recommends American and Siberian ginseng rather than the stronger, Asian ginseng. The most highly prized of all ginsengs, American ginseng once grew wild in many parts of this country, including Maine, Arkansas, and Wisconsin. Today, however, it is fairly endangered, so don't look for it in your local nursery or even in the wild.

The older the root, the better. As the plant ages, the active ingredients become more concentrated in the root.

Valued in China for thousands of years for its energy-boosting qualities, Siberian ginseng (often called eleuther) is also a favorite in Russia, where millions of people take the root daily. Siberian ginseng isn't a true ginseng (it's not in the Panax species), but it exhibits many of the same properties. The Russian Olympic weight lifting and running teams have used it to increase endurance and performance. Dozens of studies on Siberian ginseng conducted in the 1960s and 1970s, though considered sloppy by many, did support its antifatigue effects and its ability to enable you to work better longer. Proofreaders, for example, were more effective in their work after taking 1½ dropperfuls of Siberian ginseng tincture daily for 30 days. However, Dr. Kamhi emphasizes that it is not a stimulant, just a hedge against fatigue.

How to use it. Though you can buy capsules and tincture, says Dr. Kamhi, one of the best ways to use American ginseng is to buy a dried root from a well-stocked health food store. Cut off a ¼-inch piece and place it under your tongue. Though the root is hard at first, it'll quickly become soft enough to chew.

"When you're using good, strong ginseng, you'll feel a change immediately," says Dr. Kamhi. If you don't, you're probably not using a very good ginseng. You can also do as the Chinese do and use it as a seasoning for soup. Add a handful of thick slices per gallon of soup, throwing it in just as you would ginger—though it adds significantly less flavor.

Siberian ginseng root is not widely available, so your best bet is to take it in tincture or capsule form. Dr. Kamhi recommends taking 10 drops of tincture three times a day or a 1,000-milligram capsule twice a day.

Suma (*Pfaffia paniculata*)

This shrubby ground vine is native to the Amazon basin and has been used for generations in South America as an all-around tonic. The indigenous people call it Para Toda ("for all things") and also use it to treat cancer and rheumatism. Japanese residents of Brazil gave it the name Brazilian ginseng because of its restorative powers. It was introduced into the United States in the mid- to late 1980s, and herbalists consider it an effective adaptogen, meaning it helps restore balance in the body.

You probably won't find the raw root, says Dr. Kamhi, but many health food stores stock teas, tinctures, and capsules. As well as pepping up your energy levels, suma is also helpful for joint aches and pains. In Brazil, the herb is used as an aphrodisiac—as are many energy-boosting herbs. An Italian study showed that male rats given extracts of suma were significantly more sexually active than those that didn't get it.

How much? An appropriate dosage recommended by Dr. Kamhi is a 300-milligram capsule three times a day.

Licorice (*Glycyrrhiza glabra*)

Used as an herbal remedy for centuries, the dried root of the licorice plant has a sweet, musty flavor that most people either love or hate. Licorice is known for its soothing and clearing effect on the throat, and singers often chew it to keep their voices clear. The root has also received attention for its beneficial effect on gastric ulcers. The Chinese have used it as an energy tonic for centuries.

Glycyrrhizin, a major component of licorice, is 50 times sweeter than sugar, which explains why the herb is used so often in candy, chewing gum, and baked goods. The fact that glycyrrhizin foams in water has been put to good use by brewers, who use it to increase the foam on the head of a glass of stout.

Licorice is an especially good herb for women. It can ease both PMS and menopause symptoms, possibly because it contains compounds that mimic estrogen. It also helps stimulate the body's adrenal hormones, which may explain why it helps in cases of adrenal exhaustion. Herbalists theorize that being under stress for a long period of time can wear out of the adrenal glands, according to herbalist and author Douglas Schar of Washington,

More Zzzs, More Zip

"Being stressed is exhausting," says herbalist Aviva Romm, a certified professional midwife, executive director of the American Herbalists Guild, and author of *The Natural Pregnancy Book*. To increase your energy, find a way to relax and get more sleep.

Lavender, chamomile, lemon balm, passionflower, and motherwort are among Romm's favorite calming herbs. Take any of them as a tea or a tincture an hour before bedtime or whenever you feel stressed. They'll sedate you, but they'll also take the edge off your stress and help you get the rest you need.

For lavender, chamomile, or lemon balm, drink one to four cups of tea daily. A nice blend is ½ teaspoon each of chamomile and lavender blossoms plus 1 teaspoon of

D.C., and London, who has a Diploma in Phytotherapy (the medical use of herbs) and is a member of the College of Practitioners of Phytotherapy in England. Once they're worn-out, the glands fail to produce the "get up and go" hormone, adrenaline. Since licorice is an adrenal gland tonic, Schar adds, it helps the gland do what it's supposed to do.

How much? In a letter to the *New Zealand Medical Journal*, Riccardo Baschetti, M.D., a retired medical inspector in Padua, Italy, wrote of his having tried licorice for his chronic fatigue syndrome. Although his condition had persisted for nearly 2 years despite numerous other treatments, he claimed it cleared up within days after his having taken 2.5 grams of licorice in about 2 cups of milk a day. Licorice tea is easily available and tastes very sweet.

lemon balm leaf per cup of hot water. Cover and steep for 10 minutes, then strain. Or take ½ to 1 teaspoon of tincture up to six times a day.

For passionflower or motherwort, take ½ to 1 teaspoon of tincture up to six times a day. While these herbs can be taken regularly, a break every 3 or 4 weeks is advisable, says Romm.

A soothing herb bath also beats stress, says Romm. Add some essential oil to the water and shut the bathroom door so the soothing vapors don't escape. Romm's bathtime picks include lavender, spearmint, rose geranium, rosemary, and lemonrose. You could also wrap the herbs in a piece of cheesecloth and tie the homemade bag around the faucet so the hot water runs through it.

Kava Kava (*Piper methysticum*)

When stress is part of your everyday life, you can forget how to relax. When that happens, you enter a vicious cycle where sleep is hard to come by and you never feel truly refreshed or invigorated. "An herb that helps you relax, so long as it doesn't sedate you excessively, will actually make you feel more energy once you're rested," says Dr. Mulligan. For keeping anxiety at bay and helping you get the rest you need, kava kava fills the bill nicely.

A member of the pepper family, kava kava has been used for thousands of years by the South Pacific islanders of New Guinea, Samoa, Hawaii, and Polynesia to relax the body and mind. The root of this swamp-loving plant is so much a part of the culture that a whole ceremony has been developed around it in Fiji, where visiting dignitaries are served a special drink made from kava root mixed with coconut milk. The effect is swift: an instant sense of well-being and calm without any drowsiness. Scientific studies have proven that kava does indeed decrease anxiety significantly better than a placebo.

How much? When drunk as a beverage, the spicy herb has a temporary numbing effect on the mouth, lips, and throat. Although kava is traditionally used as a tea in the countries where it grows, in the United States it's typically taken as a capsule. Dr. Kamhi suggests 100 milligrams three times a day. If you need extra help sleeping, you can take 300 milligrams about an hour before bedtime.

Maca (*Lepidium meyenii*)

The Andean root called maca is becoming more and more popular in the United States. That's probably because of its reputed ability to enhance libido and improve male potency. As far back as the 16th century, the Spanish conquistadors in the Peruvian highlands fed maca to their domestic animals to deal with fertility problems associated with high altitudes. It's also a great all-around tonic herb, which is why it's known as Peruvian ginseng.

"It's one of those power boosters," says Dr. Kamhi, "and very good for women to take."

Marketed in the United States as a natural alternative to Viagra, maca now appears in health food stores with labels suggesting that it will help you lose weight, have more sex, improve stamina, and beat the blues. Though scientific research has been minimal at this point, maca is certainly nutritious, with high levels of iron, calcium, natural compounds that enhance the production of sex hormones like estrogen and testosterone, and a complement of minerals. The root's aphrodisiac qualities were confirmed for the first time in 2000 in a study involving mice and rats. Basically, the mice that received a purified extract of the root had sex more often than mice that didn't get the extract, certainly one indicator of enhanced energy.

How much? Dr. Kamhi recommends a 500-milligram capsule of dried root twice a day or 10 drops of tincture twice a day.

Codonopsis (*Codonopsis pilosula*)

Although it's not related to ginseng, codonopsis is often referred to as poor man's ginseng because it costs much less. It's an important plant in traditional Chinese medicine. The dried root of this perennial—a lovely plant with blue bell-shaped flowers—is known as dang-shen in China, where it's used to treat weakness and fatigue as well

Safe Use of Herbs and Essential Oils

Herbs are generally safe to use, but caution should always be taken with anything you ingest. To be on the safe side, pregnant and lactating women should not use any herbs without consulting their physicians. For the rest of you, here some guidelines.

Ashwaganda (*Withania somnifera*). Do not use with barbiturates because it may intensify their effects.

Asian ginseng (*Panax ginseng*). May cause irritability if taken with caffeine or other stimulants. Do not take if you have high blood pressure.

Chamomile (*Matricaria recutita*). Very rarely, can cause an allergic reaction when ingested. People allergic to closely related plants such as ragweed, asters, and chrysanthemums should drink the tea with caution.

Ephedra or ma huang (*Ephedra sinica*). Do not use if you have high blood pressure, glaucoma, heart problems, diabetes, or thyroid disease. Don't use if you are taking medication for asthma. Ephedra may increase the action of prescription drugs. Do not take regularly for more than 7 days or exceed a single dose of 8 milligrams.

Guarana (*Paullinia cupana*). Long-term use of excessive amounts is not recommended because it stimulates the nervous system. Can irritate the gastrointestinal tract.

Kava kava (*Piper methysticum*). Do not take with alcohol or barbiturates. Do not take more than the

as vertigo, anemia, and many other conditions. When taken as a decoction—meaning the tough root is simmered in water to release its healing power—this slightly sweet root is believed to restore Chi, the Chinese term for "vital energy."

Scientific research has been limited, though studies do

dose recommended on package. Use caution when driving or operating equipment, as this herb is a muscle relaxant.

Lemon (*Limon citrus*) oil. Do not use more than 3 drops in the bath. Avoid direct sunlight because this oil can cause skin sensitivity.

Licorice (*Glycyrrhia glabra*). Do not use if you have diabetes, high blood pressure, a liver or kidney disorder, or a low potassium level. Do not use daily for more than 4 to 6 weeks because overuse can lead to water retention, high blood pressure caused by potassium loss, or impaired heart and kidney function.

Nettle (*Urtica dinoica*). May worsen allergy symptoms, so take only one dose a day for the first few days.

Rosemary (*Rosemarinus officinalis*). In therapeutic amounts, may cause excessive menstrual bleeding. Considered safe when used as a spice.

Rosemary oil. Do not use if you have hypertension. Do not use if you have epilepsy, due to the powerful action on the nervous system.

Spearmint (*Mentha spicata*) oil. Don't use more than 3 drops in the bath.

Yerba mate (*Ilex paraguayensis*). Not recommended for excessive or long-term use because it can stimulate the nervous system.

suggest that dang-shen helps strengthen the immune system, increase red blood cells, stimulate the nervous system, and contribute to overall energy.

How much? You might have to check several herbal suppliers to find codonopsis in tincture form, but it is available. Take ¼ to 1 teaspoon three times a day, says

Schar, and stick with it, as it may take several months before you feel a pronounced energy boost.

Rosemary (*Rosmarinus officinalis*)

Few herbs are surrounded by quite as much delightful lore as the rosemary plant. Because of its reputation for strengthening the memory, it has become a symbol of fidelity, accompanying bride and groom down the aisle throughout history.

In her 1930s book *A Modern Herbal*, the writer and herbalist Maud Grieve quotes an old-time herbalist's advice to "take the flowers . . . binde it to thy right arme in a linnen cloath and it shale make thee light and merrie." Both calming and stimulating, rosemary is often prescribed by herbalists for psychological tension.

A 1998 study at the University of Miami tested rosemary's stimulating claims on 40 adults, 30 of whom were women. They were exposed to 3 minutes of aromatherapy with either lavender or rosemary. The lavender group showed increased drowsiness, while the rosemary group showed decreased frontal alpha and beta power in their brains, suggesting increased alertness.

How to use it. Herbalist Gayle Eversole, Ph.D., a professional member of the AHG and founder and director of the Creating Health Institute in Granite Falls, Washington, has all the proof she needs. As part of her consulting work, Dr. Eversole found herself working with a group of Boeing Company employees who complained of a midafternoon slump as they sat at their computers. "One simple thing I suggested was to put drops of rosemary essential oil on a cotton ball and place the ball on their desk so they would be continuously inhaling the aroma," she said. It worked like a charm, chasing off those workday blahs and helping the workers feel more awake.

Schisandra (*Schisandra chinensis*)

For women with hectic schedules, schisandra (sometimes spelled schizandra) is one of the very best herbs for maintaining energy, says Schar. A building block of traditional Chinese medicine, schisandra has been valued as an energy tonic for hundreds of years.

Schisandra is a woody vine that belongs to the magnolia family. The medicinal part of the plant is the fruit—shiny red berries with a taste that somehow manages to be sweet, sour, salty, hot, and bitter all at the same time. This unusual confluence of flavors accounts for the plant's Chinese name, *wu-wei-zi*, meaning "five taste fruit." Laboratory tests, conducted mostly in China, support its ginsenglike reputation for chasing away fatigue.

Schisandra also improves poor nerve function and reduces chronic coughing and night sweats. One way it works is by enabling the liver, which stores excess glucose as glycogen, to release that energizing substance into the blood, where it can work more effectively, says Schar. It also increases circulation to the arms, legs, and heart. If that's not enough, schisandra is thought to stimulate the brain and the spinal cord, revving up reflexes.

"This is a gentle herb," says Dr. Eversole. "It will adapt to you and encourage your energy to shift."

How much? Take two 500-milligram capsules in the morning and two in the evening, but don't expect overnight zip; it takes several weeks to reach full effect. You also may be able to find dried schisandra berries in Asian markets or in your health food store. The herb is also readily available as a tincture or tablet. The dosage for these forms is 1 to 6 grams of dried berries a day or 2 to 4 milliliters of tincture, divided into two portions, morning and evening, Schar says. To measure milliliters, use a dosing syringe or spoon, available at pharmacies.

Ashwaganda (*Withania somnifera*)

Ashwaganda is an Indian herb that has been fundamental to the ayurvedic healing tradition in that country for centuries. A member of the nightshade family (along with the more familiar potato, tomato, and eggplant), ashwaganda is sometimes referred to as Indian ginseng.

In India, all parts of the plant are used: the berries to thicken milk, the twigs to brush teeth. For therapeutic purposes, though, it's the roots that matter. As well as being prescribed in India for a whole litany of complaints from arthritis to heart disease, ashwaganda is prized as a general tonic to promote strength and stamina. The increased sense of energy many people feel after taking ashwaganda for even a few days often leads to heightened libido.

Research on ashwaganda seems to indicate that the herb has antistress properties similar to ginseng's. Tests have also shown that it protects rats from stress-induced stomach ulcers and enables mice to swim longer. Other studies have focused on ashwaganda's antioxidant properties and its beneficial effect on the immune system, a particularly important finding for those of us on the far side of middle age. As we grow older, immune function often falters, making us more vulnerable to infection and age-related diseases. By boosting the body's immunity, ashwaganda may actually slow the aging process.

Ashwaganda has an earthy odor and flavor that is, to say the least, an acquired taste. Fortunately, you can find ashwaganda in many health food stores in both capsule and tincture form.

How much? A recommended dosage is two 500-milligram capsules of nonstandardized extract morning and night, says Schar.

Vitamins and Other Supplements

One afternoon on her way home from work, Carolyn has a few rare minutes to spare. She has, almost blessedly, missed the usual traffic snarls.

Racing down the list of errands she can fit into these precious bits of time, she notices the little health food store she drives past almost daily.

Maybe it's time to stop. She used to take a multiple vitamin supplement, along with a few milligrams of iron. Somehow, the bottles got pushed to the back of her kitchen cabinet like so many outdated spices. Surely the supplements, too, are outdated.

She zips into the parking lot. It won't take more than a couple of minutes to pick a multivitamin, she figures.

Inside, she quickly spots the vitamins and minerals aisle. But she isn't prepared for what she sees. On one side, the shelves are stacked with multivitamins and single vitamins like E, C, and B_6. There are vitamins with minerals like iron and zinc, and minerals in bottles of their own. There are naturals, synthetics, chelated products. And doses range from micrograms to milligrams and more.

On the other side of the aisle hangs a sign: "For Energy." Underneath are dozens of other supplements, like the hormone melatonin. Carolyn thinks that one has something to do with sleep. But some of those other names: NADH, coenzyme Q_{10}, alpha-lipoic acid? They sound like something straight out of chemistry class.

Desperate for something to help her fatigue, Carolyn debates whether to grab one of the multis or an armload of supplements and hope for the best. As she instinctively glances at her watch, her muscles tighten. She has to pick up the kids and get dinner on the table—fast.

She leaves the store empty-handed and more confused than ever. Even shopping for vitamins is a physical and emotional drain!

Nearly half of us pop dietary supplements, according to a survey by the National Center for Health Statistics and the Centers for Disease Control and Prevention. Among the most common reasons for taking them? To increase energy or improve performance.

We're trying to squeeze more out of our 24 hours. And we're willing to pay to do it. We buy up to $10 million in supplements every year.

We're also reaching for plenty of products beyond the typical multi, says Barbara MacDonald, N.D., a naturopathic physician in Portland, Oregon, who specializes in women's health.

"I've had people come in with a suitcase full of supplements," she says.

When Dr. MacDonald helps her patients sort through the boxes and bottles, about three-quarters of the supplements get tossed. Some may contain ingredients that are inappropriate for them, such as the stimulant herb ephedra (also known as ma huang). Others just don't suit a woman's needs.

It's okay to supplement, Dr. MacDonald says, but you first need to talk to your doctor about other causes of fatigue, such as a thyroid condition and depression. Then you need to think about what you're trying to accomplish, she says, instead of reaching for the supplement of the moment.

In fact, many of us can benefit from vitamin, mineral, and other dietary supplements beyond even the popular herbals, says Richard A. Kunin, M.D., a nutritional specialist in San Francisco. He believes many women have marginal deficiencies of vitamins and minerals not detected in standard blood tests or physical examinations.

Why? Too many of us simply aren't eating right, Dr. Kunin says. We're on perpetual diets, skimping on calories and missing out on many nutrients. To compensate, Mother Nature dials down energy production.

"Vitamin and mineral deficiencies are characterized by a drop in energy production, a sense of malaise, and fatigue," Dr. Kunin says. We may not develop full-blown deficiencies or related diseases, such as scurvy from too little vitamin C, he says, but we won't feel at our best either, especially when we're running from sunrise to sundown.

Think of supplements, then, as a nutritional insurance policy, says Mary Ellen Camire, Ph.D., professor of food science and human nutrition at the University of Maine at Orono. They're not replacements for a poor diet or lack of exercise, however. Foods contain many beneficial nutrients that science is only beginning to understand.

Still, many products are safe to try, Dr. Kunin says.

If you combine them with other energy-boosting strategies—such as exercising, rooting out sources of stress, and eating a balance of fresh vegetables and fruits, whole grains, fish and lean meats, and low-fat dairy products—you may be able to leave fatigue in the dust.

To make the most of your few spare shopping moments, here's a look at some safe bets in the energy field as well as a few products to avoid. Most can be found in supermarkets and drugstores as well as health food stores.

Vitamin Basics

The Food and Drug Administration doesn't regulate dietary supplements like vitamins and minerals, which means it also doesn't approve them for safety or efficacy. Some things to look for include the following:

Daily Values. These are general guidelines set by the Food and Nutrition Board of the National Academy of Sciences to help avoid over- or undersupplementing. Talk to a registered dietitian or a nutritionally savvy physician before you customize a supplement plan that exceeds label recommendations.

USP. It stands for United States Pharmacopeia, and its presence on a product is an indication the product is pure and contains the listed nutrients. Also, look for an expiration date to be sure the product is potent.

Store brand or name brand? Synthetic or natural? In most cases it doesn't matter, says Mary Ellen Camire, Ph.D., professor of food science and human nutrition at the University of Maine at Orono. Folic acid, the synthetic form of a B vitamin, is one exception. We absorb and use the synthetic form more easily.

Fillers. Some women may be allergic or sensitive to stabilizers, starches, cellulose, and additives in supplements.

Chelated. This simply means a mineral is bound to another substance to hasten its absorption. There's little evidence that chelated materials work better, and they can cost five times more.

Managing with Multis

Thirteen vitamins and more than three dozen minerals help us turn food into energy and the tissues that compose our bodies. Each works in a slightly different way, however, and we need them in varying amounts to feel our best every day.

Unless you're eating at least 1,600 calories a day, you probably aren't getting all the nutrients you need for optimal health from your food, especially during your childbearing years, says Joanne Larsen, R.D., L.D., a registered dietitian in Seattle.

One of the simplest, safest, least expensive ways to supplement is with a multiple vitamin and mineral combination that contains 100 percent of the Daily Values (DV) or Dietary Reference Intakes (DRI) set by the Food and Nutrition Board of the National Academy of Sciences, Dr. Camire says.

In general, says Dr. Camire, look for a product that contains at least the vitamins A, C, and the B complex as well as minerals such as calcium, chromium, copper, iron, manganese, selenium, and zinc.

How much? Dr. Kunin says it's safe to take up to 10 times the DV for most vitamins and twice the DV for all minerals except iron, magnesium, and potassium. "For many people," he says, "the recommended amounts are not enough."

Bet on the B Complex

When it comes to energy, the B-complex vitamins—thiamin, riboflavin, niacin, B_6, B_{12}, folic acid, pantothenic acid, and biotin—are most often linked to peak mental and physical performance.

They help us turn carbohydrates into the blood sugar that fuels our cells, muscles, and brains. And each works a bit differently, says Dr. Camire.

Vitamin B_6, for instance, helps form neurotransmitters, the nerve chemicals that send messages to our brain. B_{12} makes red blood cells that contain iron-dense hemoglobin and deliver energizing oxygen to our cells. Folate, or folic acid, makes amino acids, the building blocks of life-sustaining protein.

We get the Bs in beef, chicken, and other animal foods and in whole grains, such as breads and cereals.

Suboptimal levels of the Bs may contribute to fatigue. And they're difficult to assess through standard blood tests. "The science isn't there yet," she says.

In one study, 12 people with untreated chronic fatigue syndrome had lower levels of B_6, riboflavin, and thiamin than did 18 healthy people.

We also need more Bs as we age. For example, as the years go by, our bodies absorb less B_{12}, even when we eat foods rich in it. If you're vegetarian or if you eat little meat, you're also at risk for lowered B_{12} levels. A deficiency can lead to pernicious anemia, where you don't make the red blood cells you need and so feel headachy and miserably fatigued.

Then there's folic acid, vital to energy stores. "Lots of folks run low on folic acid, unless they take it in a vitamin," Dr. Kunin says. Even the Nutrition Board has upped its recommendation for folic acid over the years, to 400 micrograms.

Folic acid helps our bodies make new cells, and it works with B_{12} to form hemoglobin—the oxygen-carrying protein of our red blood cells. We also can develop anemia if we get too little folic acid. And women of childbearing age should take folic acid even before they become pregnant because studies show it helps prevent neural tube defects such as spina bifida.

How much? The Bs work together, like a well-rehearsed orchestra. So choose a multiple B product that supplies 25 to 100 percent of the Daily Value for each vitamin. Rebecca Wynsome, N.D., a naturopathic physician in Seattle, sometimes gives B_{12} injections to patients with diminished levels of the vitamin to offset anemia. The injections deliver the vitamin more quickly than a capsule or liquid sold in health food stores. For others, she recommends supplementing with at least 50 milligrams of B_{12}, riboflavin, B_6, and niacin. This is higher than the DV for niacin (35 milligrams), so check with your doctor before taking that amount. Too much niacin may cause flushing, itching, and other side effects.

C: The Energy Vitamin

The benefits of vitamin C extend far beyond boosting our immune systems. It's a powerhouse for fueling us through our day, Dr. Kunin says. Along with a host of other attributes, vitamin C makes a substance in our bodies called carnitine, which our muscles need to burn fat for energy.

C also is a potent antioxidant that boosts immune function and energy by enabling the adrenal glands—which sit atop the kidneys and regulate the stress hormone adrenaline—to work properly, says Dr. Wynsome.

We get vitamin C in fruits such as oranges and vegetables such as broccoli. But studies show that only about 17 percent of us eat the recommended five fruits and vegetables we need daily for optimal health and vigor, and one in four Americans doesn't even get the recommended DV of 60 milligrams of vitamin C.

When we're low on C, "it shows up in very short order as malaise and a lack of energy," Dr. Kunin says.

In a study of 400 healthy people conducted by researchers at Arizona State University in Tempe, 30 percent showed levels of vitamin C low enough to cause fatigue. Another 6 percent had levels indicative of vitamin C deficiency.

How much? Many nutritionally oriented physicians, including doctors Kunin and Wynsome, recommend up to 1,000 milligrams daily, even more under conditions of physical stress and illness. The safe upper limit set by the Food and Nutrition Board is 2,000 milligrams. Try dividing the doses in two to keep blood levels of C steady all day. One possible side effect of such high doses is diarrhea. Cutting back on C, without cutting it out, can help.

Mind Your Minerals

Choosing vitamins is as easy as ABC. But choosing minerals is a bit trickier, says Larsen.

That's because minerals are more dependent on one another for their actions. As with a seesaw, if you take too much of one, you may tip another out of balance.

Minerals are critical for good health and energy. They repair tissues and bones, ferry oxygen to cells, guard your nervous system, and even help your muscles contract.

Yet feasting on zinc, for example, may blunt your levels of copper. Gulping down iron tablets daily may sink zinc levels. To get around that, select a multivitamin with minerals and follow the Daily Values on the label, suggests Larsen.

Key players on the energy field include the following:

Pump iron. If we're going to work out in the gym or even haul that load of laundry up and down the stairs, this mineral is a must.

Iron, as part of the hemoglobin in your blood, helps to taxi oxygen to every cell and muscle within you, including your brain. Just like a nice, deep breath, oxygen makes for energy.

Menstruation and our own propensity to avoid calorie-dense red meat puts women at risk for low iron levels. If we get too little iron, we become pale, tired, and listless.

The Consequences of Low Iron Levels

Iron deficiency anemia causes that knocked-down, dragged-out feeling. It occurs when you don't have enough iron to make hemoglobin, the blood cells that deliver energizing oxygen to your muscles, lungs, and brain. But you don't need full-fledged anemia to suffer the consequences of low iron.

Probably 8 to 10 percent of women are borderline anemic, says Jere Haas, Ph.D., director of the division of nutritional sciences and professor of maternal and child nutrition at Cornell University in New York. In these cases, suboptimal stores of iron go undetected by standard hemoglobin tests and generally are ignored during physical checkups, says Dr. Haas. Yet they can drain you without your even knowing it, especially since deficiencies come on slowly, with no clear symptoms.

You're most at risk for deficiency in your childbearing years—when you lose blood through menstruation—or when you skimp on iron-rich meats in your diet. Before menopause, choose a supplement containing 18 milligrams of iron a day; go for one with 9 milligrams or less at menopause and after. If you're anemic, your doctor may prescribe more. (Be aware that too much iron is just as dangerous as too little, as it increases your risk for cardiovascular disease and cancer.)

If you suspect you're marginally iron-deprived, ask your doctor for a hemoglobin test. If your levels are 13.5 or below, ask for a serum ferritin test, which counts iron in the liver and detects marginal levels more precisely.

Premenopausal women need 18 milligrams of iron a day. At menopause, however, look for a multiple with no more than 9 milligrams—or none. Too much iron can lead to cardiovascular and other problems. Meats, fish, and poultry contribute the most iron, but legumes, enriched grain products, and eggs are also good sources. If you eat little or no meat, you may need an iron supplement, so check with your doctor.

If your doctor recommends an iron supplement, the most common form is ferrous sulfate. You should avoid taking more than 18 milligrams a day unless a blood test indicates that you're anemic.

Copper up. This mineral helps you store and release iron so your oxygen-ferrying blood can fuel your tissues and muscles. Copper is abundant in fish, shellfish, legumes, nuts, peanuts, raisins, soybeans, and spinach.

But—surprise, surprise!—most of us come up short on copper. Dr. Kunin says 7 out of 10 of us don't get enough. When he prescribes supplements, "many people wake up more alert, and some bound out of bed," he says.

Look for a multi with a DV of 2 milligrams copper, but no more than 9, the safe upper limit set by the Food and Nutrition Board.

Beware when buying: One study showed many multis contain a copper compound called cupric oxide, which our bodies don't absorb. Look for copper sulfate or cupric sulfate on the label.

Think zinc. Found in every cell in your body, zinc has garnered headlines in recent years as a cold treatment and possible player in improving short-term memory.

But zinc might also help on the energy front by smoothing out the highs and lows in your insulin and blood sugar levels. A shortage can leave you feeling sluggish, fatigued, lethargic. And zinc—most abundant in meat and oysters—is one mineral you're likely to lack.

Studies show that exercising hard over long periods zaps zinc stores. Long-term endurance training, such as running, significantly lowers zinc levels in women and men and can result in decreased endurance.

When choosing a multi with zinc, look for 15 milligrams, the DV. The safe upper limit: 30 milligrams.

Magnesium? Maybe. When our diets are less than perfect—sound familiar?—we may not get enough magnesium.

It's found in green vegetables, nuts and seeds, dried beans, and whole grains, but in tiny amounts. So getting enough from food alone is difficult.

Magnesium turns your food into energy and keeps your muscles and nerves humming on even the most harrying of days. One study of 16 healthy men deprived of sleep and asked to exercise on stationary cycles showed that those given 100 milligrams of magnesium performed better than those who received none.

Diuretics, some antibiotics, and some cancer medicines increase your loss of magnesium, as does excessive alcohol use.

When shopping for magnesium in a multi, choose one with 100 milligrams; few have more than that. The DV is 400 milligrams, and the safe upper limit is 700 milligrams, but more than 350 milligrams in a supplement may cause diarrhea. To get more than 350 milligrams without the uncomfortable side effects, try eating more magnesium-rich foods.

As with other minerals, it's possible to get too much magnesium. If you've got heart or kidney problems, check with your doctor before supplementing with the mineral.

Chromium: It's not on your bumper. You may have heard about this mineral, as it's gained quite a reputation as a weight-loss aid. Although studies in that regard are mixed, people who take chromium supplements often say they're more energetic, says Harry G. Preuss, M.D., professor of medicine at Georgetown University Medical Center in Washington, D.C.

That may be because chromium, found naturally in foods such as apples, sweet potatoes, brewer's yeast, and molasses, helps you burn carbohydrates for fuel. Doctors suspect it also helps keep your insulin and blood sugar levels in check so you're less likely to feel shaky or fatigued on a blood sugar roller coaster.

Dr. MacDonald often recommends 200 micrograms a day of chromium picolinate, the form people absorb best. The DV is 120 micrograms; the safe upper limit is 1,000. But check with a doctor before choosing a supplement with more than 200 micrograms.

Supplement Savvy

Beyond the alphabet soup of vitamins and minerals on the health food or pharmacy shelves, you almost need a dictionary—or an encyclopedia—to work your way through some of the newest supplement labels marketed to the fatigued masses.

These supplements have varying claims to fame. Some build strength or muscle; others reenergize your days or help you sleep better at night.

However, there are no Daily Values for other over-the-counter supplements. So start with a quality health food store or ask a nutritionally oriented physician for advice, says Barbara S. Silbert, D.C., N.D., a chiropractor and naturopathic physician in Brookline, Massachusetts.

If you self-supplement, follow product labels carefully for dosages.

Here's a look at what's out there.

CoQ$_{10}$. A coenzyme is a vitamin-like molecule that boosts metabolism, which is the release of energy from food. Coenzyme Q$_{10}$, or ubiquinone, is an antioxidant and an essential part of the mitochondria, or energy centers in your cells. There, it creates adenosine triphosphate, or ATP, the fuel your cells run on.

Though most of us aren't deficient in CoQ_{10}, levels do decline with age.

The energy spin comes from studies suggesting that combining CoQ_{10} and a high-potency multivitamin and mineral supplement may help women with chronic fatigue syndrome.

In heart patients who may be deficient in CoQ_{10}, the supplement seems to work by improving the heart's ability to contract and to use oxygen.

Because it's an antioxidant and an energizer, Dr. Silbert sometimes prescribes CoQ_{10} to help women overcome fatigue from cancer and its treatments.

CoQ_{10} is sold as capsules or soft-gels of 10 to 200 milligrams. Dr. MacDonald recommends 30 milligrams a day, particularly for athletes, to replenish energy stores. There are no known side effects. Discuss supplementation with your doctor if you are taking the blood thinner warfarin (Coumadin).

NADH. Preliminary studies on NADH, or nicotinamide adenine dinucleotide, suggest this supplement may rekindle energy for women with chronic fatigue syndrome or even the garden-variety, I'm-just-tired kind of fatigue, says Dr. Preuss. Like CoQ_{10}, the supplement is a coenzyme and contributes to the high-grade cell fuel ATP.

In a preliminary study at Georgetown University School of Medicine in Washington, D.C., 26 women with chronic fatigue syndrome took 10-milligram capsules of NADH or a placebo (worthless pill) daily for 4 weeks. Thirty percent of those taking NADH reported renewed vigor, compared with 8 percent of those who had swallowed a placebo.

Though the study was small and more work is needed, that's a significant finding, says Dr. Preuss, one of the researchers. Chronic fatigue syndrome is "the worst of the worst fatigue," he says. So the study holds promise—even for those of us who just need a jolt around midafternoon.

Women with chronic fatigue syndrome should consult a physician before taking NADH. Otherwise, try 10-milligram capsules once a day, preferably with food. Some women report feeling better after about a week, Dr. Preuss says.

The supplement is considerably more expensive than a vitamin tablet, he notes. But it appears safe, with no known side effects. Nervousness and loss of appetite have been reported in the first few days of supplementing, and the supplement may cause stomach upset.

Looking for an even better pick-me-up? Dr. Preuss suggests taking CoQ_{10} along with NADH. Try one for about a month and then add the other. Or take them together.

DHEA. It's dehydroepiandrosterone, a hormone produced by the adrenal glands, which sit just above the kidneys.

"It's the bank account of energy," says Dr. Wynsome, who sometimes prescribes DHEA along with cortisol, another hormone related to energy, if salivary tests show a woman's levels are depleted. When we're drained of these hormones, we may indeed be exhausted. And their levels drop as we age.

But Dr. Wynsome does not recommend over-the-counter DHEA supplements for women. Here's why: When we take DHEA without a physician's guidance, our bodies may churn out too much estrogen or testosterone. That could increase our risk for breast cysts, aggressive behavior, or even cancer, Dr. Wynsome says. And too much of the predominantly male hormone testosterone in women may cause facial hair and acne.

Sometimes, patients tell Dr. Wynsome they're using a number of supplements, including DHEA, and experiencing these typical side effects without being aware that the hormone is to blame.

So stay away from it, says Dr. Wynsome, unless you're under a doctor's care.

Melatonin. More than 20 million Americans turn to melatonin each night in hopes it will bring them slumber.

The irony is that there's no clear evidence the supplement, often a synthetic version of the hormone we produce naturally, actually helps us get a better night's sleep, says Nancy Fishback, M.D., of the Sleep Disorders Center at Sentara Norfolk Hospital and Eastern Virginia Medical School in Norfolk, Virginia.

We get our melatonin from the tiny, pinecone-shaped pineal gland in the brain. The gland goes into production around dusk, sending melatonin into the bloodstream, where it reaches its peak levels around 2 A.M. Melatonin is critical to a sound night's sleep. And it can help with jet lag, Dr. Fishback says, by adjusting our internal clock. "But no one knows what an effective dose is," she says.

One study of eight adult hospital patients in intensive care, where sleep deprivation is common, showed that melatonin treatments improved both the duration and the quality of sleep and may help reset the biologic clock.

But Dr. Fishback says the research isn't strong enough to recommend we turn to melatonin supplements when we're tossing and turning at night. "It will probably be an important drug someday," she says, "once more is known about its actions."

You should take melatonin only under the supervision of a knowledgeable medical doctor because with many medical conditions it may lead to adverse effects. It may also interact with prescription medications.

Creatine. If you work out at a health club, this supplement probably sounds familiar. Creatine is popular with athletes bent on building muscle and enhancing performance. It comes from animal foods, such as meat and fish, and 95 percent of it gets tucked away in your muscles, where it mixes with phosphate and becomes a backup source for ATP.

Creatine can provide quick bursts of energy for running or strength training, according to a report from Tufts University, and supplements may reduce muscle fatigue, so you can exercise longer. But it probably won't do much if you're looking for a burst of midafternoon energy—even if you're at the gym, says Melvin H. Williams, Ph.D., professor emeritus of exercise science at Old Dominion University in Norfolk, Virginia, and coauthor of *Creatine: The Power Supplement.* And there are potential side effects.

One survey of college baseball and football players at the University of Washington in Seattle who used creatine showed they experienced muscle cramps, diarrhea, and weight gain when they regularly took doses higher than the recommended 2 to 5 grams per day. And nine male baseball players who took creatine as part of a study at Old Dominion University gained 5 pounds in just the first week. Not exactly a side effect most women want.

Bottom line, says Dr. Williams: If you're interested in serious strength training, creatine may be worth a try. But forget about it for a daily energy boost.

Alpha lipoic acid. Ever wonder where a 2-year-old gets her energy? This is where. Unfortunately, by the time we're 40 or 50 (and trying to deal with that 2-year-old daughter or granddaughter), our supply is sorely depleted. Yet without this mighty antioxidant, we wouldn't have enough energy to push the button on the remote control, let alone master those calendars jammed with activities and obligations, says Bert Berkson, M.D., Ph.D., of Las

Cruces, New Mexico, and author of *The Alpha Lipoic Breakthrough*.

Lipoic acid helps metabolize carbohydrates, fats, and amino acids, jump-starting everything from our brains to our toes. Lipoic acid also keeps other energy-providing antioxidants like vitamin C and vitamin E in the body longer.

We get lipoic acid from many foods, including liver, broccoli, and spinach. Yet they don't contain much. Consider: We'd need to put away 200 pounds of spinach to take in one-third of the recommended daily amount.

"You really need to supplement if you want the high energy you need," Dr. Berkson says.

It appears to be safe, says Dr. Berkson, but he suggests talking to a nutritionally oriented physician or nutritionist before trying it. Look for capsules or tablets from Germany or Italy, which, Dr. Berkson says, are of the highest quality.

Try 100-milligram tablets three times a day, preferably with meals. Prepare to feel an energy boost in about 10 days.

Women with diabetes can safely supplement with 600 to 1,000 milligrams a day, says Michael Janson, M.D., of Arlington, Massachusetts, and author of *Dr. Janson's New Vitamin Revolution*. But make sure you tell your doctor.

One caveat: Lipoic acid supplements may lower B vitamin stores, so if you're taking it, supplement with a B-50 complex.

Carnitine. This substance also powers the cell's inner engine, the mitochondrion, by carrying fatty acids across cell membrane so they can be burned for fuel.

Carnitine-containing foods include avocados, red meat, and dairy products, but the body also makes its own supply. The trouble is, production fizzles as we age.

Research shows carnitine supplements may safely enhance your physical performance, Dr. Janson says. There also is evidence that carnitine may benefit people with chronic fatigue syndrome.

Dr. Kunin used carnitine to treat leg cramps in one female athlete. The woman was also taking valproic acid, a medication for mood disorder that interferes with the natural production of carnitine. She experienced leg cramps after cycling on a stationary bike for only 2 minutes at 90 percent of peak performance. After 1,000 milligrams of L-carnitine daily for one month, she was able to bike for 23 minutes without cramping

For general fatigue, Dr. Janson suggests 1,000 milligrams of L-carnitine daily, divided into two doses. It's most often sold as tablets. Do not take the "D" form because it may cause muscle weakness; doses above 2,000 milligrams may cause mild diarrhea.

Moving into Energy

Carolyn confides to her best friend, Beth, "Some days I barely have the stamina to drag myself to bed at night." They're sitting in a restaurant near their offices, indulging in a rare, relaxing lunch instead of chewing french fries in front of the computer.

"You should join my aerobics class," Beth says.

"Ha!" Carolyn laughs. "Getting through the day is enough of an effort. Why would I want to tire myself out even more?"

"You'd be surprised how much more energy you have when you work out," her friend replies.

Carolyn wonders if Beth is right. Could going to a step class make waking up in the mornings easier? Could lifting weights make her energy slump less noticeable? While she doesn't know how she'd fit it into her schedule, she likes the idea of using exercise to let out some of her tension and stress.

A week later, during a particularly exhausting afternoon at work, she calls Beth. "Where do I sign up for your aerobics class?"

Carolyn has the right idea. Moving more really will give us more energy to do those things that seem so hard: dragging ourselves out of bed before the sun comes up, carrying an overflowing laundry basket up the stairs, surviving a stressful day at work.

Exercise—whether it's a formal aerobics class or a heart-pumping dig in the garden—not only helps our bodies by burning fat and strengthening our bones and muscles but also stimulates our metabolism, improves our sleep, enables us to avoid illness and chronic disease, and keeps us mentally healthy.

You know that drained feeling you get when you're fighting a cold or the flu yet continuing to do the million things you do every day? If you exercise, you're less likely to get sick in the first place because your workouts wake up your immune cells, which attack and kill bacteria and viruses. And because working out keeps us healthier overall, we'll have more energy not only now but in every stage of life. Researchers say the decline in health that occurs between the ages of 30 and 75 is due only partly to aging. It can also be blamed on lack of exercise.

The problem for most women: Being told to exercise is like being told to eat Brussels sprouts. We know it's good for us, but it's hard to swallow. Fewer than 10 percent of Americans exercise four times a week, and fewer women than men get a regular workout.

In a survey of 2,002 people, more than half of them women, 23 percent said that nothing—not their doctors' advice, pleading from family, or access to workout facilities—would increase their physical activity. Among those who *do* start an exercise routine, half quit within a year.

Maybe we stop because we think exercise has only one purpose: to help us lose weight. When we don't drop 10 pounds after a month of aerobics, we throw in the towel.

What Exercise Does for You

To reduce your risk of disease in the future, it's important to be more active now. Here's how staying active
helps prevent disease.

- Weight-bearing exercise—like weight lifting,
  step aerobics, walking, and even gardening—
  puts tension on muscles and bones and forces
  your body to compensate by increasing bone
  density.
- Exercise reduces the risk of breast cancer among
  pre- and postmenopausal women.
- Moderate to intense exercise for a half-hour
  helps lower blood glucose levels and blood
  pressure, decrease insulin resistance, improve
  cholesterol levels, decrease body fat, and prevent
  type 2 diabetes.
- Brisk walking, jogging, swimming, biking, aerobic dance, and racquet sports improve the
  way your blood clots, lower blood levels of
  artery-clogging triglycerides, and raise the blood
  level of HDL ("good") cholesterol, thereby
  lowering your risk of heart attacks and heart
  disease.
- Researchers suspect that exercise lowers the risk
  of stroke.
- Exercise reduces the risk of some forms of
  cancer, such as colon cancer and cancers related
  to obesity.
- Strength training improves digestion and lowers
  LDL ("bad") cholesterol levels.
- Stretching and abdominal crunches help prevent
  back pain.

We're also more confused than ever about what it means to be in shape, says exercise physiologist and personal trainer Risa Olinsky, M.A., owner of Classic Fitness, Inc., in Maplewood, New Jersey. Too often we think fitness equals a sculpted body, but size has nothing to do with it, she says. She knows slender women with low fitness levels and overweight women with strength and endurance.

Something else we need to get over: feeling like we haven't had a good workout unless we're completely exhausted. Exercise should produce a pleasantly tired feeling, not make you want to collapse on the couch.

Once you begin to feel your own energy and strength, it's hard to let go. Ask 49-year-old Martha Coopersmith, founder of The Bodysmith Co., a personal training firm in New York City. She runs 15 to 20 miles a week, works out twice a week with her own trainer, and knows her own strength, which usually lets her do anything she has to.

"Few things are too heavy for me to lift," she says, whether she's moving furniture in her living room or carrying several heavy grocery bags.

She views exercise as something we're *meant* to do, and she's right. In fact, research suggests that we're actually hardwired for it. The nervous system has a control center that regulates energy. This biological control system keeps a balance between the calories we take in and the energy we expend. After taking in more calories, we naturally want to move. And, Coopersmith reminds us, when we move more often, we gain better health, strength, and confidence.

"For some people, exercise is like religion," Coopersmith says. "It's something they believe in, it gives them a calm, and they can always rely on it to make them feel better."

Research supports the anecdotal evidence. A small study of cancer patients suffering from fatigue found that aerobic exercise clearly reduced their exhaustion and gave them more energy for daily activities. Another study found further evidence: People with chronic fatigue syndrome who did regular aerobic exercise felt more energized than those who didn't.

Although her clients are usually skeptical at first, Olinsky says, they usually tell her they feel more energetic once they start a workout program. After a few weeks of lifting weights and walking, they report feeling more rested in the morning and less drowsy in the evening.

"When you start exercising, you realize you have energy you didn't know you had," Olinsky says.

Exercise's Edge

It's hard to believe that tiring yourself out actually gives you more energy. Here's how it works.

When you do a significant amount of aerobic activity and lifting weights, your muscles adapt and increase in size. Your heart and vascular system, which transports blood, become more efficient, improving the delivery of oxygen. That makes it easier to get up and go when you have to. You also produce more of the hormone testosterone, which is necessary to build and maintain muscle. The more muscle you have, the higher your metabolism, and so the cycle continues.

If you think of metabolism as the flame of a gas stove that's always lit, food is fuel for the fire, and exercise is the control valve. Every time you turn up the heat by walking or jogging, your body works to provide more energy for the workout by breaking down carbohydrates and fats, delivering oxygen to your tissues, and storing more glycogen and triglycerides in your muscles. Over time, the cycle becomes more efficient, and you feel like you have more energy.

Also, simply being stronger makes it easier to get through the day.

After age 40, you begin to lose 6 to 8 percent of your muscle every 10 years. The good news: It takes only 2 months of strength training (at 40 minutes, three times a week) to gain back 20 years of muscle. If you can't lift weights that often, you'll benefit from even a fraction of that time.

Exercise's Calm

Besides all the physical benefits, a great workout simply makes you *feel* good. And when you feel good, you have the energy to accomplish your day-to-day tasks—and then some.

Let's start with the ring of the alarm clock. After exercise, your muscles are more relaxed, and you get a better night's sleep. Come morning, you feel more refreshed.

As for the rest of the day, you're often confronted with difficult situations: fighting traffic during your commute, working overtime, arguing with the kids to get their homework done. Confronting these circumstances may cause physiological reactions known collectively as the fight-or-flight mechanism: perspiration, accelerated respiration, increased heart rate and blood pressure. When your body's systems return to normal, you can be left feeling both emotionally and physically drained. But you don't have to.

When you exercise regularly, a similar physiological reaction takes place—your heart rate increases, you perspire, and so on—but when you're finished exercising, you're not left with that wiped-out feeling that often lingers after a stressful day. Instead, you can feel calm and even rejuvenated. That's because regular exercise trains the body to better handle the physiological reactions (the heart gets stronger, the respiratory system functions more efficiently) and to recover from them more quickly.

The best part: Once your body is conditioned to respond in this way, it'll do so in response to a variety of stimuli, not just in response to exercise. So when faced with a difficult situation, chances are you won't feel so exhausted and will regain your energy more quickly. Exercise can even be better than meditation in getting rid of anxiety. During exercise, studies show, your brain releases endorphins, the feel-good hormones that produce the "runner's high" you hear about. Consistently exercising also increases levels of your resting hormones, such as serotonin, dopamine, and acetylcholine. When levels of your resting hormones are higher, it's easier for you to relax because they keep your heart rate and blood pressure low.

The mind–body connection exercise provides probably also has something to do with improved physical feeling. When you use your muscles, you're focused on that activity: putting one foot in front of the other, breathing rhythmically, getting the aerobic moves right. You clear your mind. And along with the release of endorphins, that results in a heightened state of alertness when you're finished. It might even be as good as psychotherapy in lessening depression, while it can also enhance your creativity and imagination.

Exercise also gives you something you don't always have in the rest of your life: control. You control your health and fitness when you work out regularly. *You* control how far you walk, how long you swim, how fast you run. *You* define what success feels like, whether it's a 5-minute mile or bench pressing your weight. That sense of control spills over into the rest of your life, providing you with more confidence and thus more energy.

An Energy Plan

The official recommendation from the Surgeon General is to exercise 30 minutes on most or all days of the week.

All together now: gro-o-o-oan! But working out doesn't have to equal traditional exercise, and it doesn't mean you have to do it for 30 minutes continuously. In fact, all you may need to do is increase the time you already spend on certain activities, such as dancing. Here's how to create your own energy-enhancing program.

Figure in your fitness level. If an aerobics class is just too much for you to jump into right now, start with lower-impact activities, such as walking or gardening. You might be surprised to learn that many of the routine things you do every day provide you the same workout as walking or aerobics. In half an hour, a 150-pound woman burns 136 calories walking briskly, 221 calories doing aerobics, and 272 calories playing singles tennis. Compare that with the activities below, whose calorie-burning powers are based on the same 150-pound woman. Although the number of calories burned isn't the issue—you're trying to increase energy, not lose weight—burning a certain number of calories assures that your metabolism goes high enough to provide increased energy.

Shoveling snow: 204 calories
Outside carpentry, such as building a fence: 204 calories
Scrubbing the floor or mowing the lawn: 187 calories
Dancing to disco, country-and-western, or polka music: 187 calories
Gardening: 170 calories
Trimming shrubs with a power trimmer: 119 calories

Even more good news: Researchers found that women usually work out longer and burn more calories doing these kind of activities because their motivation comes from simple enjoyment instead of weight loss.

Choose a variety. For the energy of strong muscles, endurance, and flexibility, you need strength training, stretching, *and* aerobic activity. Women who skip strength training and work only their cardiovascular system eventually lose upper body strength.

Of course, the big question is "Will strength training make my muscles bulky and unattractive?" The experts' answer: a resounding no. Want some proof? Marilyn Monroe, a feminine icon in her own right, lifted weights.

Promise yourself half. If you really think you can't make it through the entire 30 minutes of exercise, tell yourself you'll walk, swim, or inline skate for just 15 minutes. Chances are, once you get going, you'll keep going. Even if you don't finish, at least you got a start—and maybe you'll do more tomorrow.

Break it up. If you don't have a 30-minute block, break up your workout into three 10-minute walks throughout the day, or add lifestyle activities, such as walking to work, taking the stairs, and parking as far away from the door as possible.

"You can even work while you work out," Coopersmith says. "I put a problem in my head before I go running. By the end of my run, I often have a solution."

Please your personality. If you like the outdoors, hike in the summer and cross-country ski in the winter. If you like exercising in privacy, pop an aerobics tape into your VCR. If you enjoy being around others, join a walking group.

If none of these please you, think about what you liked to do as a kid, Coopersmith says. If you loved roller skating, try inline skating. If you were a gymnast, join an adults' gymnastics class. Chances are, you'll still enjoy doing it.

To recruit others for your workout, start a before-work, lunchtime, or evening walking group with friends or coworkers. Or organize your own sporting events with neighbors, and set up a volleyball net or play soccer at your next picnic.

Get the beat. Put together a tape of songs that move from a slow to a fast beat and reserve it for your walk. The opportunity to listen to great music will probably get you out of the house. And once you get moving, Barry White will warm you up and Gloria Estefan will help you to step up the pace.

Put on the pressure. Sign up for a charity walk or join a sports team. When you know you've set a specific goal, no matter the size, you're more likely to stick to your workouts.

Take toys with you. Buying some "toys" might just get you moving. You might try a heart rate monitor when you walk, a medicine ball for some different strength work at

Energizing Stretches

You can do these stretches at your desk or sitting in any chair. Hold them between 15 and 30 seconds, with deep breathing throughout, says exercise physiologist and personal trainer Risa Olinsky, M.A., owner of Classic Fitness, Inc., in Maplewood, New Jersey.

Stretch your neck and shoulders to relieve tension headaches. Sit very erect on the edge of your chair and look straight ahead. Lace your fingers behind your head as if you are lying back in the sun. Take a deep breath. Exhale, slowly tuck your chin to your chest, and gently press your head down and forward. Inhale as you lift to the starting position. Repeat three times.

Stretch and relax your back. Sit on the edge of your chair with your feet flat on the floor, hip distance apart. Relax your arms to your sides. Take a deep breath. Tuck your chin to your chest. Begin to exhale and slowly roll forward until your chest is resting on your thighs (as if

home, a stability ball for abdominal crunches, resistance bands to work your legs and arms, or a chinup bar hung in a doorway in your home.

Bring the dog along. Taking Skeeter on your walk will do more than provide good company. He might rely on the workout so much he'll give you that extra nudge on days you try to skip.

Train Swedish-style. In Sweden, they take the routine out of exercise with an interval trail training called "fartlek." Go as fast as you can for as long as you feel comfortable; then slow down. When the urge hits, do situps and pushups—whatever keeps you moving and having fun, even if it means skipping your way through 30 min-

your body is folded in half). Breathe deeply from this position and, as you exhale, uncurl your back to a straight-up position. Repeat three times.

Wake up fatigued arms, neck, and shoulders. Straighten your right arm and cross it over the left side of your body at shoulder height, with your palm facing back. With your left hand, hug your right upper arm, gently pressing it against your body. Keep your right elbow soft and slightly bent. Breathe deeply. Rest and change sides to repeat.

Loosen up tight hamstrings and calves. Sit up tall at the edge of your chair with your feet flat on the floor. Extend your right leg straight out in front of you, keep your heel on the floor, and flex your toes toward the ceiling. Relax and place both hands on your left thigh, take a deep breath, and lean forward as you exhale. You will feel a stretch in the back of the straight leg.

utes. If you're having fun, you'll be more motivated to finish your workout. This type of interval training also increases your fitness level, which helps with energy.

Change the scenery. Yeah, yeah, if you have to walk by your neighbor's pink flamingos again, you'll puke. So hike in the woods or walk around the mall.

Congratulate yourself. Don't let small achievements go unnoticed. They're proof that you're making progress. Thank yourself for working out when you're less tired after grocery shopping or when you can walk, garden, or play tennis longer than usual.

The Energy Workout

For optimal energy, you need a regular program that combines cardiovascular activity, flexibility training, and strength and toning exercises. To get started, try this general fitness workout designed by personal trainer Olinsky.

To know if you're working at the right level, rate how you feel on a perceived exertion scale of 1 to 10. One is easiest; it's how you feel sitting down, watching television. Ten is hardest—how you would feel sprinting uphill. Work on a perceived exertion level of 5 or 6.

Be aware that not every exercise is right for every person. You need to listen to messages your body sends you. Of course, you should check with a health care professional if you have individual limitations, like back or knee problems, that may affect your ability to try these exercises.

Have cardiovascular fun daily. Work in 30 minutes of cardiovascular fitness every day by choosing an activity that's enjoyable—something you want to do. You might try family bike rides, singles tennis, cross-country skiing, swimming at the beach, a brisk walk with a friend, inline skating, or ice skating. Whatever you do, start out at a comfortable speed and gradually increase intensity within

5 minutes. You should break a light sweat and be slightly breathless but still able to hold a conversation.

Strength train two to three times a week. Always start your strength workouts with at least a 5- to 8-minute cardiovascular warmup. This will increase heart rate, break a little sweat, and increase muscle temperature, preparing the muscles to work harder. You will need a few sets of dumbbells, in weights ranging from 3 to 10 pounds. Which one you use will depend on your fitness level and the body part you are working. Different muscle groups require different weights. Your biceps (the front of the upper arm) might need a 5-pound dumbbell, while your triceps (the back of the upper arm) might require a 3-pound one. And remember: To get stronger, your muscles need time to rebuild and adapt to the stress placed on them during the strength work, so space your workouts throughout the week, leaving at least a day between them.

Use weights that you can lift slowly and steadily for one set but that are too heavy to lift more than 15 times. Lifting anything lighter won't build muscle. When you're able to do more than 15 reps, you can either increase to a second set with the same weight (with a rest of 30 to 45 seconds in between) or increase the weight slightly and maintain a one-set program. Move at a comfortable pace without stopping too long at the top or the bottom of each movement. Exhale during exertion.

• *Squats.* Looking straight ahead, stand with your feet slightly wider than shoulder-width apart, toes turned slightly outward. Keep your shoulders back and extend your arms forward for balance. Slowly bend your knees and drop your hips toward the floor as if you are going to sit on a stool. Stop when your thighs are parallel to the floor, so that your knees are at a 90-degree angle. Keep looking straight ahead; don't look down. Return to an upright position, being careful not to lock your knees. Make sure your feet stay flat on the floor throughout the movement. To intensify this exercise, hold a dumbbell in each hand and keep your arms by your sides.

• **Chest fly.** Lie on your back on a flat bench, a piano bench, a step bench, or even a narrow ottoman. Bend your knees and place your feet parallel on the bench (or place your feet flat on the floor on the sides of the bench). Allow your spine to relax without arching or being pressed down. Hold a dumbbell in each hand, with your hands alongside your chest. Your palms should be facing each other. Inhale and slowly open your arms to the sides, with bent elbows, until you feel a slight stretch across your chest. Don't go so far that you lose control of the weights. Do not straighten your arms. You should be able to see your hands in your peripheral vision. Exhale as you return your arms to the starting position.

• **Overhead press.** With a dumbbell in each hand, stand with your feet shoulder-width apart. Start with your arms bent and the dumbbells at your shoulders. Keep the arms close to your body. Take a deep breath; with your palms facing each other, press the weights straight overhead, exhaling as you press upward and being careful not to lock your elbows. Do not lean back as you lift. Inhale as you lower the weights back to your shoulders.

• **Row.** Put your left knee on a bench or the seat of a sturdy chair and bend over so your back is straight and parallel to the floor. Rest your left hand in front of you on the bench or chair and extend your right arm toward the floor. With a dumbbell in your right hand, pull your hand up until it almost reaches your armpit, keeping your arm close to the body. Lower the arm straight toward the floor and repeat. When you finished a set with one arm, repeat with the other arm.

• **Triceps press.** Sitting on a chair with a weight in your right hand, raise your right arm overhead. Your elbow should be bent and your palm should be facing your ear and close to it. The weight should be behind your head. Support your right arm with your left hand as you lift the weight overhead and exhale. Lower it back behind your head again; inhale, keeping your palm facing your ear. Try to keep your elbow fixed in one place as you raise and lower the weights. Concentrate on keeping your abdominal muscles tight to keep your back aligned. When you finished a set with one arm, repeat with the other arm.

• *Biceps curls.* Stand with your feet shoulder-width apart and knees slightly bent. Hold your weights at your sides with your palms facing forward. Bend your arms as you slowly raise the weights to your shoulders, exhaling and making sure your elbows stay close to your sides. Lower the weights back to your sides and inhale. This movement can be done with both arms at the same time or alternating arms.

• *Abdominal crunches.* Lie on your back with your knees bent and your feet flat on the floor. (A carpet or mat will make this more comfortable.) Your back should be in a neutral position, neither arched nor pressed to the ground. If you have one, place a soft squeeze ball about the size of a soccer ball between your knees and hold it there to help stabilize your knees. Lace your hands behind your head for gentle support and take a deep breath. Exhale as you slowly lift your upper torso a few inches off the floor. If you are using the ball, gently squeeze it with your knees at the same time. Focus upward; don't tuck your chin. This will help keep your head aligned with your spine. Lower yourself as you inhale, keeping your back as straight as possible.

Stretch after you work out. Stretching not only boosts your energy level but also helps prevent injury by releasing the tension you've placed on muscles during your workout. Be sure to stretch right after your exercise session, because that's when your body is most pliable. Muscles and other connective tissues in your body are like rubber bands—if you pull too hard when they're cold, they snap.

Here's a good stretching exercise for your back and hips. Lie flat on your back and bend your knees so your feet are flat on the floor with your toes pointing forward. With your arms extended outward and your palms face-down on the floor, inhale deeply. As you exhale, slowly drop both knees over to the left side, keeping your feet and shoulder on the floor, and your knees together. After holding for 30 to 45 seconds, bring your knees back in to your chest and repeat on the other side.

Finding Energy
the Alternative Way

Carolyn stares blankly at her computer screen. Eyes fixed on the cursor, her mind ticks off the endless to do list that dominates her every waking moment—stop at the grocery store for peanut butter on the way home, print out a fall release schedule of new software, order prescriptions for her mother, mend Michael's soccer uniform.

"Hey, are you still on this planet?" Carolyn's head snaps toward the voice. It's her coworker Beverly, delivering an inventory printout. Beverly always has a spring in her step and a sparkle in her eye, even though her job is just as demanding as Carolyn's and she has three kids. What's her secret?

Yoga, comes Beverly's simple answer. She first took it up 10 years ago when her children were small and her fatigue overwhelming. It gives her time away from the whirl of life, a chance to recharge—plus, it's great for muscle tone.

"You should try it," she tells Carolyn.

But Carolyn isn't sure yoga is for her. Her mental image of a yoga class is a New Age salon filled with lithe,

Gumby-like creatures contorting themselves into impossible poses. Beverly assures her that isn't the case and scribbles the name of her teacher on Carolyn's desk pad. "What can you lose by trying a few classes?" she calls as she turns to go.

Carolyn sits at her desk feeling like the poster girl for 21st-century overload. With fatigue threatening to become *the* defining feature of her life, she decides she's ready to try anything—even yoga.

She's not alone. Alternative health treatments like yoga have gained wide acceptance in this country largely because these techniques seem to work where more conventional methods don't. The proportion of Americans using alternative therapies like massage, herbs, vitamins, energy healing, and homeopathy rose from about 33 percent in 1990 to more than 42 percent in 1997. In addition, in 1997 Americans spent more than $27 billion on these therapies, more than we spent out of pocket for hospital costs.

Alternative therapies may tend to be better for chronic conditions like fatigue, allergies, and stress because they treat the root cause of illness rather than just the symptoms, says Mark Stengler, N.D., director of natural medicine at Personal Physicians clinic at La Jolla, California, associate clinical professor at the National College of Naturopathic Medicine in Portland, Oregon, and author of *The Natural Physician*. For instance, if you have mild allergies, a naturopathic doctor wouldn't just suggest you pop a decongestant. He'd evaluate your digestive system, where mucus and histamines are made, then propose a treatment plan aimed at correcting the problem underlying the stuffiness in your head.

Approaches differ, yet all alternative therapists suggest that good health depends upon a natural energy balance of all body systems, known as *homeostasis*, says Dr. Stengler. Every cell has a perfect energy balance, he says, just as the body as a whole has a perfect energy balance. Too much stress disrupts this equilibrium and may cause all manner of illness. Most alternative medical theories are based on the concept that vital life energy—called Chi—flows throughout the body along invisible zones called meridians. Balanced, freely flowing Chi generates good health, says Dr. Stengler, while sluggish, blocked, or over-stimulated Chi is a sign of poor health.

"Chi flows through the body like blood," he says. "There is an electrical charge to the body, and treatments that strengthen and balance energy flow have been shown for hundreds of years to improve health." Exactly *how* they work is still a mystery. But the same can be said for facets of conventional medicine.

Tap, Tap, Tap Your Way to Energy

Some naturopathic physicians believe the thymus, an endocrine gland located behind your breastbone, plays an important role in your energy levels because two of the body's energy meridians run through it. The thymus is large in infancy and starts shrinking after puberty. This results in a slow decline of immunity throughout adulthood.

So by tapping your breastbone firmly—21 times is the recommended number—you may stimulate the thymus and enhance energy (according to Chinese medicine theory). "Don't pound your chest like Tarzan," says Mark Stengler, N.D., director of natural medicine at Personal Physicians clinic in La Jolla, California, associate clinical professor at the National College of Naturopathic Medicine in Portland, Oregon, and author of *The Natural Physician*. But do tap decisively with the tips or flats of four fingers or a loose fist.

As for Chi's relation to energy, "we each experience energy in our own way, but one thing is certain: Energy flows," he says. "It circulates consciously and unconsciously throughout the body on a physical, emotional, and mental level."

One sign of the popularity of alternative therapies is their accessibility. You need look no further than the nearest YWCA or community health club for yoga. Chiropractic offices are nearly as prevalent as gas stations. And even corporate offices bring in massage therapists for on-the-job treatments.

Although their popularity has exploded in just the past decade, most alternative therapies have ancient roots. Our interest may have brought them back into public consciousness, but in truth, when it comes to finding energy the alternative way, "everything old is new again."

Yearn for Yoga

Yoga stems from Hinduism, one of the oldest religions on the planet. It's a discipline that engages your mind as well as your body, with roots going back about 5,000 years. Many women practice yoga to find personal meaning in life and in the process gain energy, vitality, and an improved sense of well-being.

Yoga is about the balance of your physical, mental, and spiritual states. Its purpose, according to yoga philosophy, is to get your physical body under control so the more perfect "inner you" can emerge. Yoga practitioners learn to breathe properly and strengthen their bodies through exercises known as poses or postures.

"Because yoga connects the body and the mind, it tends to energize women more than aerobics," says Dawn Braud, director of the fitness center at Woman's Hospital in Baton Rouge, Louisiana, and an exercise physiologist.

Unlike forms of exercise that involve strictly your body, yoga has a psychological aspect that encourages you to mentally "let go" of the day's burdens, says Braud, giving your mind a chance to recharge as well.

Yoga is also a stress reducer, which makes it an ideal workout, says Braud.

"What the mind has forgotten, the body remembers," she says, but after the deep relaxation of yoga, these stressors melt away, leaving you refreshed.

The beauty of yoga is that it is diametrically different from our on-the-go lives. No multitasking here. Instead, yoga rooms are quiet and serene, and the art requires mindful concentration if you're to get the poses right.

As a result, says Braud, most women leave a yoga class feeling lighter, a little less burdened.

At the core of yoga philosophy is the belief that we have three bodies—the physical body, the astral body (or mind), and the causal body (or pure spirit), reached through meditation. While each can function separately, they are intimately interrelated, so to know your whole self, you must have an awareness of all three bodies. When you do, you reach a state of self-actualization where, yogis say, you'll realize your profound connection to the universe and its abundant energy.

The beauty of yoga is in its versatility. You can focus on the physical, the spiritual, the psychological, or a combination of all three. Unlike traditional forms of exercise, which tend to be goal-oriented, yoga is a process. Your awareness is focused on what you're doing and how it feels. With the "happy pose," or triangle, for example, your focus is on the stretch in your legs, chest, and arms.

The pose works like this: Stand with your legs about a yard apart, the right foot pointed forward and the left foot comfortably turned out. Bend from your waist to the left, resting your left hand on your left ankle or calf, and extend your right arm straight up over your head. Feel the stretch in your neck as you look straight ahead or up to the sky. As you hold this pose, notice how strong your legs feel against the ground and the way your chest opens up, bringing in energizing oxygen.

Too often, women are intimidated by the idea of an exercise class, believing they're not fit enough to even join. Not so with yoga, says Braud. "You can start at any level of fitness," she says, "and yoga will meet you where you are." Then, as you improve with practice, you graduate to more difficult postures.

Unlike exercise classes where you learn the routine and repeat it, yoga is an ongoing learning process. You can learn a pose, then refine it, says Braud, moving on to more and more challenging variations as you advance.

And unlike many ultrahip exercise trends to hit the market, "yoga is not about looks," says Braud. Classes are filled with people of all shapes and sizes. A totally non-judgmental discipline, "yoga has you focus inside," she says, "and you can be in any body to do that."

Realizing the benefits of yoga requires some dedication. Braud recommends working out three to five times a week for 20 to 30 minutes.

Within that brief time, the meditative aspect of yoga can put you back in touch with who you are, both emotionally and spiritually, Braud says. "In today's society, we tend to become disconnected from our mind and spirit," she says, "which makes us far too vulnerable to other people's expectations, one of the biggest energy drainers around."

To find a yoga class: Holistic health centers and YWCAs are a good place to start. Or check out www.yogasite.com, which has a state-by-state directory of teachers. This site also lists workshops and retreats across the country. To receive general information on what to look for in a yoga instructor, send a self-addressed envelope with postage for 2 ounces to the American Yoga Association at P.O. Box 19986, Sarasota, FL 34276, or check out its Web site, www.americanyogaassociation.org.

Massage the Energy In

Strong fingers knead the tops of your shoulders, then glide up your neck. The tension in taut muscles begins to dissolve, and before long the soreness that always seems to lurk at the base of your skull starts melting away. As the pressing and stroking continue, stress evaporates from every muscle group, leaving you limp with relaxation.

There are approximately 100 different methods of massage therapy, the majority performed with various hand strokes. Part of Chinese medicine for more than 4,000 years, massage in some form has been part of Western healing since the fourth century B.C., when it was endorsed by the Greek physician Hippocrates.

Massage not only feels exquisite but also has healing and energizing properties.

It's gaining widespread acceptance today as scientists document the effects of touch through biochemical changes in the brain and body, says Donna Mack, R.N., director of the Center for Health and Restoration at Mercy Medical Center in Baltimore.

Blood chemical tests of patients done before and after a massage show an increase in T cells, which bolster the immune system, and endorphins, the body's natural painkillers and destressors, says Monica Haynes, R.N., certified massage therapist at the Center for Health and Restoration at Mercy Medical Center in Baltimore.

Apart from manipulating muscles to relieve stress and promote relaxation, massage therapy helps to energize people through touch, says Haynes. "Touching is an intimate act," she says. "Whether we're rocking a baby or giving someone a hearty handshake, when we touch another person, something happens between us." Massage therapists know that touch can convey the therapeutic emotions of caring and concern, she says, and some believe that touch can help release blocked emotions, allowing the patient's body to revive itself.

At the very least, the total relaxation that massage affords allows your body to repair the daily damage done to it by stress, Mack says, noting that most women come to her center seeking stress reduction. "As energetic as women's lives are today, we get sapped of energy, largely through stress," she says. "Massage allows women to go into a very deep state of relaxation. From that state, the body can heal and reenergize itself."

Whether you prefer a traditional European method or some form of Oriental manipulation, all types of massage can take you to that healing state of relaxation, says Mack. In her opinion Swedish massage—the type most commonly performed—with its long, gliding strokes, works best for stress reduction. Its guided strokes tend to promote a more nurturing, loving massage, she says, more so than a treatment-type massage that pinpoints a particular discomfort.

"You can tell that a woman's stress has been dramatically reduced when she steps out of a massage room looking like a limp dishrag," says Mack. And although it sounds counterintuitive, such deep relaxation is actually quite energizing.

To find a qualified massage therapist: Many hospitals and health clubs employ massage therapists. The American Massage Therapy Association (AMTA) can refer you to a qualified therapist in your area. You can call AMTA's Find a Massage Therapist national locator service at (888) 843-2682 or visit its Web site, www.amtamassage.org/findamassage/locator.htm.

The Energizing Effect of Water

Hydrotherapy is an age-old form of healing that uses water in a variety of therapeutic ways. To practice it at home, use a handheld shower massage attachment to run warm water up and down your arms and legs for 15 seconds. Follow with 15 seconds of water that's as cool as you can comfortably stand. (Cold is too shocking and stimulating to the system.)

The warm water soothes and relaxes, while cool water stimulates your immune system, says Mark Stengler, N.D., director of natural medicine at Personal Physicians clinic in La Jolla, California, associate clinical professor at the National College of Naturopathic Medicine in Portland, Oregon, and author of *The Natural Physician*.

The contrast between warm and cool improves circulation and provides overall stimulation. If you continue this alternating shower for 5 minutes, says Dr. Stengler, you'll feel a decided spike in your energy level.

If you live near a hydrotherapy clinic, Dr. Stengler suggests you try a total relaxation treatment. Showers and tubs customized with high-powered jet sprays can wash away tension from stressed-out muscles. Initially, you may feel a tad tired from your aqua pummeling, he says. But within a few hours, you'll experience a marked energy rebound.

Our Feet and Hands: Fonts of Energy

Grab your big toe. Press your thumb firmly into the bottom tip. Hold for 90 seconds. Repeat with the opposite foot. In a few minutes, you should start feeling your weariness lifting. Believe it or not, pressing the flesh in certain areas of your feet and hands—following a system of alternating pressure techniques called reflexology—may reduce fatigue, leaving you refreshed and alert.

Reflexologists believe the body's bioelectrical energy, or Chi, flows in meridians throughout the body. Every organ falls along one of these meridians, which end at the tips of our fingers or toes. According to this healing art, which dates back to at least 2330 B.C., the soles of the feet and the palms of the hands represent a map of the body. Applying pressure to the correct point on these extremities sends an energy signal that stimulates a specific organ, such as the brain. Anything that unblocks the energy meridians into the brain will quickly increase energy, says Marcia Aschendorf, N.M.D., a board-certified naturopathic physician who runs a private clinic in Cincinnati and who is also executive director of the International Academy of Naturopathy.

By clearing any blockages that stop Chi from circulating freely throughout the body, this signal, say reflexologists, also strengthens and balances your body's vital energy flow.

"Reflexology can quickly alleviate fatigue by restoring mental alertness and reducing tension," says Dr. Aschendorf.

A simple example: When people wring their hands because they are sad or overwhelmed, they're instinctually employing a form of reflexology. This action brings energy into the body in times of distress, she says, noting that people often unconsciously do whatever their bodies need to feel better.

The brilliance of reflexology, Dr. Aschendorf says, is that you can practice it on yourself, in any setting, whenever your energy starts lagging. Energy is very personal, she says, and it needs to be revitalized when different events of the day sap it.

Here are two energizing exercises you can do yourself.

- For a quick energy burst, bring your hands together, fingers straight as if in prayer, and then flex the fingers of both hands so that the tips are touching with your palms a few inches apart. Tap your fingertips together for 3 to 5 minutes. For maximum energy stimulation, be sure to tap the tips, not the pads, of your fingers, Dr. Aschendorf says.

Your fingertips and the ends of your toes correspond to the brain, which controls vital life functions, explains Dr. Aschendorf. Triggering this so-called brain reflex restores vitality by directing your body to breathe more efficiently and by stimulating mental electrical exchanges.

- Make a "butterfly" with your hands by placing one thumb on top of the other. Your palms should be facing away from your body. Curl the fingers of the top thumb's hand over onto the fleshy part of your other hand under your thumb. Wherever the middle finger of the top hand falls, apply firm pressure on the opposing hand's thumb mound, pulling it slightly "just like you're milking," Dr. Aschendorf says. Do this for 90 seconds. Reverse hands and repeat.

Dr. Aschendorf says that this exercise boosts your energy by stimulating the adrenal reflexes, which govern the heart, lungs, and kidneys. You can perform a variation of this exercise in your car when you're at a stoplight, Dr. Aschendorf says. Simply press the fleshy mound of the palm below the thumb into the steering wheel, holding the pressure for several seconds and then releasing. Tapping your fingertips on the steering wheel helps, too.

Healing Powers of Homeopathy

This 200-year-old system of holistic healing is based on the idea that "like cures like." It claims to stimulate the body's own recuperative powers through remedies containing extremely small amounts of substances that, in larger quantities, would produce the very symptoms they're meant to treat.

A few conventional therapies, such as allergy desensitization and immunization, follow the same "law of similars." Because remedy extracts in homeopathy are so highly diluted, the Food and Drug Administration (FDA) does not require them to undergo safety testing. The FDA estimates that sales of homeopathic remedies are around $201 million and are growing by 20 percent a year.

Homeopaths say that, paradoxically, the more dilute a homeopathic remedy is, the greater its potential to cure. The highest potency, or most dilute, homeopathic remedies contain virtually none of the active substance, so their demonstrable efficacy seems to defy known laws of chemistry and physics. No one knows why it works, says Dr. Stengler, beyond the belief that an extract's vibration provokes the cell structure to return to normal. "Everything in nature works on a frequency," he says. "Think of your body as one big cell that receives energy vibrations. Homeopathy seeks to reestablish its system of harmony."

While there are general homeopathic remedies available in health food stores, Dr. Stengler says the most effective treatment is specific to the individual. If you're dragging through the day, a homeopath or naturopathic physician should evaluate the cause, he says, and suggest treatment uniquely for you.

State licensing requirements for such physicians vary, although most stipulate some type of medical training. To find a homeopath in your area, you can contact the National Center for Homeopathy at (703) 548-7790 or consult its Web site, www.homeopathic.org.

Before prescribing remedies for new patients, homeopaths conduct in-depth interviews designed to determine your basic physiological and psychological characteristics. These mind/body characteristics, called typologies, are important factors in prescribing the right remedies, especially for chronic conditions.

There are two basic types of remedies—single and combination. Single remedies, which contain one active substance, are generally more effective. Combination remedies, with two or more active substances, are designed to offer the greatest relief to the greatest percentage of sufferers. Each active substance is intended to alleviate a distinct symptom, with some overlap built in to ensure a higher rate of success.

Potency is indicated by a standard code, with a number indicating the number of dilutions performed and a letter indicating the ratio of each dilution. The letter "X" stands for a 1:9 dilution, while "C" indicates a 1:99 dilution.

Homeopathy is frequently used to treat fatigue and stress, says Dr. Stengler. If you can't wait to see a practitioner, here are some remedies he says work for most women.

Arsenicum. Good for mental and physical exhaustion, especially when symptoms of anxiety are present. An extremely dilute form of arsenic, this poison is extracted from metals such as iron and cobalt, then finely ground and weakened by mixing with larger and larger amounts of milk sugar. Typically, health food stores sell 30C tablets. Dr. Stengler suggests taking two tablets twice daily.

Gelsemium. Specific for feelings of drowsiness and fatigue, especially when the muscles ache as well. This is the diluted preparation of yellow jasmine. Dr. Stengler suggests taking 30C tablets, two tablets twice daily.

Phosphoric acid. This is the homeopathic dilution of the same ingredient that makes soda pop fizz. It's best used when you're so fatigued you may not be able to get out of bed. It's also good if you have a strong craving for carbonated beverages. Dr. Stengler suggests taking 30C tablets, two tablets twice daily.

Ferrum phosphoricum. Good for low energy due to iron deficiency anemia. This compound of iron and phosphorus, either of which can be deadly in large enough amounts, is diluted with milk sugar to make them nontoxic. Dr. Stengler says most widely sold formulations are 6X, and he recommends three tablets three times daily. Your doctor should monitor you with blood tests to make sure your anemia is improving.

If you try an over-the-counter homeopathic remedy, don't take it within 30 minutes of drinking coffee because the coffee may cancel out any positive effect. For the same reason, it's best not to touch a tablet; rather, shake it into the lid of its container; then drop the tablet under your tongue. If you're using a liquid remedy, shake the bottle first.

Flower Essence Energy

If you want to enjoy vigorous, blooming health, Dr. Stengler suggests flower essences, which counteract those negative emotional reactions that zap our energy.

Flower essences are specially prepared liquid concentrates made by soaking flowers in pure spring water. Each treats a specific emotion, like stress or anxiety. Developed more than 70 years ago by a homeopathic physician, Dr. Edward Bach, the essences contain specific plant energy that affects the energy balance of the person taking them.

A dose of 2 to 4 drops of an essence, taken in a glass of water or dropped under the tongue, may reset the body's emotional equilibrium, says Dr. Stengler. By restoring homeostasis, the body's natural energy balance, flower essences **restore** vitality and prevent negative feelings from leading to physical illness, he says.

Dr. Bach distilled 38 separate essences. He also created an emergency combination of flower essences he called Rescue Remedy, which Dr. Stengler suggests every woman carry in her purse.

When we're faced with sudden bad news or a stressful event, this liquid remedy may help us face the distress and emotional rebound from it, he says, by reducing fear and nervousness, two major energy siphons.

The Sound of Energy

Music touches the core of our soul. Its power transcends language, cultures, and generations. Have a cranky baby? Soothe her with a lullaby. Want to crank up your energy level? Slip in a CD of upbeat tunes.

The therapeutic effect of sound dates back thousands of years. The modern discipline of music therapy began after the world wars. Community musicians went to government hospitals to play for veterans to ease their physical and emotional traumas. The patients' responses prompted the doctors and nurses to ask the hospitals to hire musicians. Today, music is used in many hospitals to alleviate pain, induce sleep, and counteract apprehension or fear.

Almost any style of music can jazz you up or help you decompress stress, as long as it's a sound you like. But don't just be a passive listener. Making music can also boost your energy and reduce stress. So next time you need a lift or a little relaxation, try rhythmic drumming or heartfelt singing. You may be surprised by how good you feel.

Rescue Remedy contains five flower essences: impatiens (to allay impatience and irritability), star of Bethlehem (to relieve the aftereffects of fright, grief, or shock), cherry plum (to keep at bay fear of losing control and other irrational thoughts), rock rose (to calm feelings of terror or sudden alarm), and clematis (to treat daydreaming and lack of interest in the present).

Rescue Remedy is available in most health food stores. Dr. Stengler suggests 4 drops of Rescue Remedy under the tongue whenever you're faced with a traumatic irritation like an aggravating traffic jam or a fight with your boss.

Flower essences are generally safe to use under the tongue, swallow, apply to the skin, and use in the bath. However, avoid getting them in your eyes, and don't apply them to mucous membranes or abraded skin. Most flower essences contain alcohol as a preservative, so check with your doctor before using them if you're sensitive to alcohol.

Energizing Fragrances

Freshly baked apple pie. Lavender in full bloom. The powdery smell of a newborn. Certain smells make us smile; they make us feel good.

That positive feeling is the core of aromatherapy, which uses fragrant concentrated plant extracts, known as essential oils, to soothe the mind, restore balance within the body, and treat a variety of symptoms, including fatigue.

Aromatherapists believe that essential oils work on the emotions because the nerves that enable us to smell are directly linked to the brain's limbic system, which governs our emotions.

Practitioners say the active components of each essential oil give it unique therapeutic qualities. The scent of lavender, for example, is calming, while thyme is strongly stimulating.

People in ancient times used aromatic substances for medicinal, cosmetic, and religious purposes.

Energy-enhancing aromatherapy remedies include the following:

- Citrus oils. They have antidepressant and uplifting qualities, providing a pick-me-up for people with flagging energy.
- Peppermint. Invigorating and good for fatigue and depression. Three drops is the most you should use in the bath, and you should avoid getting it near your eyes. Also, do not use at the same time as homeopathic remedies.
- Frankincense. Stimulating and elevating to the mind.
- Rosemary, geranium, and basil. All are energy boosters. Rosemary has a powerful effect on the nervous system, so it's not recommended if you have hypertension or epilepsy. Don't use more than 3 drops of basil oil in the bath, and avoid it altogether if you're nursing.

Not every energizing scent works for every person, Dr. Stengler cautions. "Scent is very individualized," he says. "What may elevate one person's mood and energy level may drive another crazy."

To find an essential oil that will help ramp up your energy, Dr. Stengler suggests you sniff and react. If you draw back from a scent, it's not for you; if you draw closer, that's the right one.

Essential oils can be used externally many ways, but never apply them directly to your skin or swallow them. Use essential oils in half the recommended amount during pregnancy, and avoid using them altogether on infants and small children. Store essential oils in dark bottles, away from light and heat, and out of the reach of children and pets. When you find an energizing scent, put a few drops on a cotton ball or a wad of tissue and tuck it into your bra, between your breasts. Your body heat will cause the scent to radiate upward for a constant energizing whiff.

To keep your energy up at work or home, infuse your environment by placing essential oil in a lightbulb ring, which heats the oil and diffuses the scent throughout the area.

You can also use essential oils in a relaxing bath or energizing foot soak. No matter what you choose, your energizing oil will alleviate fatigue, Dr. Stengler says, and invigorate your entire body.

Visualize Your Way to Energy

Our minds will believe anything we tell them. So if we spend all day thinking about how exhausted we are, we'll *be* exhausted. But if we let go of those negative thoughts and emotions and see ourselves sparkling with energy, always up for life's next challenge, eventually we'll start feeling that way, says Edie Raether, a psychotherapist in Raleigh, North Carolina. That's the key to visualization: If you conceive it and believe it, you can achieve it.

"If you're not capitalizing on this tremendous power we all have to gain more energy and a better life, you're wasting a tremendous natural resource," says Raether. But don't think in terms of letters or words. Your mind is like a small child, she says; it comprehends pictures far better than words. When you visualize what you want, you need to provide a clear blueprint for the body, she says. You need "marching orders" that your unconscious mind can put into effect.

Visualization is actually a means of gaining control over our lives, she says. Too often, we move through life reacting to events, trapped in a perception of being overwhelmed. These feelings drain our energy.

The miracle of visualization is that it speaks the language of the body, says Raether, noting that the most dramatic illustration of its power has come in the battle against cancer. Anecdotal evidence collected over the past 30 years has brought visualization into the mainstream mix of cancer treatment. The American Cancer Society says that imagery may help cancer patients because it promotes relaxation and reduces stress. Although it can't cure the disease, the organization notes, it is an important technique that helps the mind influence the body in positive ways.

You should practice visualization at least once a day, Raether says, more often if possible. And you have to dispense with the negative before you can put in the positive. "You can't plant a beautiful garden in a weed-infested patch."

Begin by sitting or lying in a relaxed posture with no physical stress on your body. Close your eyes and breathe easily. Empty your mind of everyday thoughts. This means forgetting about the leak under your car, the braces your 13-year-old needs, and the silent treatment you've been getting from your boss. This, says Raether, is much more challenging than it sounds.

Focus on your breathing. As you feel yourself entering a relaxed, trancelike state, begin visualizing. The visualization should involve all of your senses—see it, smell it, taste it, touch it, hear it. "Bombard your sensory systems," says Raether. "Sensory details activate neuron centers in the brain. The more brain activity there is, the more real the visualization becomes. It's like getting all your ammunition working for you."

See yourself springing out of bed, tingling with anticipation at the glorious day stretching before you. The sun is wrapping you in a warm glow of energy. Your spine is straight, your stride confident, as you effortlessly pluck the perfect outfit from the closet. You personify energy itself

What Is Energy Medicine?

Practitioners of energy medicine believe that the human body is composed of various energy fields and that we get sick when the energy in those fields is blocked, unbalanced, or otherwise disturbed.

Therapists use a variety of techniques to balance and release the body's flow of energy. Most place their hands either on or near the patient's body. Treatments like "healing touch," or Reiki, operate on the belief that a trained practitioner can feel or sense a person's energy field. By altering "rips" or "blockages" in that person's energy field, practitioners say they can help a patient relax or heal.

Any form of touch changes your energy, as your body and the therapist's experience an energy exchange, says

as you visualize yourself moving through the day, poised and in control.

Don't limit yourself. Use your mind like a telephoto lens: Magnify your goal; see it bigger, bolder, brighter. If you want enough energy to rise at 5 A.M., work out for an hour before going to the office, distinguish yourself in your profession, help your kids with their homework, cook a healthful dinner every night, and then get romantic with your life partner, you've got to think big!

Meditate on Energy

Many cultures recognize the calming, therapeutic effect of quiet contemplation or meditation. If visualization actively puts a specific idea into motion, meditation asks you to stop, let go, and passively observe the experience of life, says Raether.

Donna Mack, R.N., director of the Center for Health and Restoration at Mercy Medical Center in Baltimore. Nurses and other healers have always known intuitively that the way people are touched can speed the healing process. The difference today, she notes, is that scientists are beginning to quantify the effect.

Several alternative therapies, including homeopathy and acupuncture, are based on energy and the ability to rebalance it for healing. Naturopaths can read a patient's life energies through a computerized biofeedback device that determines the type of stressors—like pesticide exposure or clogged internal organs—causing ill health.

Reams of anecdotal reports indicate these treatments work, but conventional science cannot yet say why.

Meditation is a self-directed practice for relaxing your body and calming your mind. It is a free-flowing experience, she says, like spontaneous artwork. As you relax into meditation, you enter an altered state of consciousness, sending your brain into a resting but aware state. Detaching, she says, helps you disconnect from the stressors of normal life, allowing your body to truly rest and recharge.

Although meditation seems simple, keeping the usual stream-of-conscious thoughts from flowing through your mind takes practice. Thoughts of dirty dishes and children's science projects will pop up on your blank mental canvas, dragging you back to the real, exhausting world. When other thoughts intrude, Raether suggests, take notice of them; then let them go.

Meditate in a quiet place with as few distractions as possible. Sit quietly in a comfortable position, preferably with your back straight. Focus your mind on your breath, on a silently repeated sound, or on a stationary object like a flower or a candle.

Focus your mind on a single thought, allowing all other thoughts to float away. Gently refocus as many times as necessary.

Practice for 15 to 20 minutes twice a day, if possible. Meditating at the same time every day helps reinforce the habit, Raether says. Many people who practice meditation say that the relaxation and focus provided by regular sessions positively affect every aspect of life, especially their energy levels, she says. Several studies show a decrease in blood pressure among people who meditate regularly.

Brush On the Energy

It may sound ridiculous, but the act of brushing your dry skin first thing in the morning could give you an instant energy lift.

It not only feels great but also stimulates the sensory nerves of the peripheral nervous system (the nerves and ganglia outside the brain and spinal cord), energizing your entire body, says Dr. Stengler. It may also improve your circulation and your lymphatic flow, the clear fluid that transports white blood cells, thus strengthening your immune system. Sloughing off dead skin cells may also help speed your body's expulsion of toxins through perspiration, says Dr. Stengler, noting that many of his clients who practice daily skin brushing report fewer ailments like headaches, colds, and flu.

To start, you'll need a natural-bristle body brush, the type available in any bath shop. Start out with medium-soft bristles. Bristles that are too stiff and hard will literally scratch your skin, and too-soft bristles are ineffective.

Once you get used to brushing, you can move on to a slightly firmer version.

You can use either short- or long-handled brushes, but a long-handled one makes it much easier to reach your back. And don't share with your loved ones. Think of this brush as you do your toothbrush, says Dr. Stengler—for personal use only. Be sure to clean your brush every few weeks with soap and water and allow it to air-dry.

Starting with your feet and ankles, brush upward in quick strokes. Work your way up to your calves and thighs, then up your torso, then up your arms from the fingers to the shoulders. Every stroke should be directed toward the heart, says Dr. Stengler. You should concentrate brushing in the lymphatic areas of your body—your inner thighs, behind your knees, under your arms—he says, to give those glands a little extra stimulation, encouraging the expulsion of toxins.

Brush the entire surface of your body, excluding your face and breasts, he says, where the tissue is too delicate for brushing.

The whole process should take no more than 3 minutes, yet it should leave you revved and reenergized. If you shower in the morning, do your body brushing in advance, says Dr. Stengler, so that any cells left behind are washed away. Some women brush their bodies before bed, finding it a good way to relax at the end of the day, he notes.

Be Thankful and Energize

An attitude of gratitude can make a huge difference in your everyday energy levels, says Raether.

In fact, there's an emerging school of thought among psychologists that promotes the power of optimism. "Positive psychology" explores how affirmative human feelings affect life satisfaction. The first positive psychology summit was held in January 2000, with the theme "Building a Positive Human Future."

Rather than feel burdened by your responsibilities, be grateful for them, says Raether. Be thankful for the mess after a party because it means you have friends. Rejoice in the piles of laundry and ironing because it means you have a family to nurture. Revel in that lawn that needs mowing and those gutters that need cleaning because it means you have a home.

Work at viewing your daily rounds as a privilege, not drudgery. "The more you practice gratitude, the more positive your life will become and the more energy you will have," she says.

And while you're at it, laugh a little.

It's impossible to be uptight when you're in the midst of a belly laugh, says Raether. Your body is totally free of anxiety and stress, building up your energy stores.

So try to see things in a humorous light as much as you can. Remember what some psychologists say: "Comedy is tragedy, plus time." Turning today's catastrophe into a giggle will make you a more energetic person, says Raether.

Play and Creativity

One sunny Sunday in February, Carolyn and her neighbor Jean take their kids to the park for a morning of snow tubing. Carolyn plans to sit at the top of the hill and supervise. But when Jean takes off on a tube, whooping her way down the slope as the kids yell encouragement, Carolyn just has to follow.

Off she goes, hair streaming, eyes tearing—and with a few delighted shrieks of her own.

Her ride lasts 30 seconds, max. But her sense of exhilaration lingers as she hauls her tube up the hill for another run.

And another. And another.

By afternoon, Carolyn has taken dozens of runs. And while she's physically exhausted, she feels more energetic than she has in weeks.

On this bright winter's day, she's learned a powerful lesson: Play isn't just kid stuff. And it can be extremely energizing.

It's true that children are masters of play. Whether they're into block towers, elaborate tea parties, or skipping rocks across a pond, they view the world as a vast playground, and play as vital to life as breathing.

Once we become grown-ups, though, the playground shrinks. Balancing the checkbook takes precedence over checkers; cleaning house, over playing house. An anthill, once a thing of mystery and awe, is now just a sign to reach for the bug spray.

We lose touch with what it means to play—to do something for no payoff, no purpose, other than to have fun. Worse, the less we play, the less we use our creative energies. It's that "all work and no play makes Jane a dull girl" thing.

Women may be particularly "play deficient," says Lenore Terr, M.D., clinical professor of psychiatry at the University of California, San Francisco, and author of *Beyond Love and Work: Why Adults Need to Play*. All that working and mothering and nurturing makes it hard to stay awake, much less play.

But if we want more *zing!* in our lives, more spring in our step, more light in our eyes and fire in our bellies, we must make time to swing on the jungle gym of our minds. Therein lies vitality, the unseen generator of mind, body, and spirit.

Are We Having Fun Yet?

Play is not just an activity. It's a state of mind.

And while there's virtually no research on adult play, the few scholars who do study it say that it is, quite literally, soul food.

"Play is a refuge from ordinary life, a sanctuary of the mind, where one is exempt from life's customs, methods, and decrees," says Diane Ackerman, Ph.D., visiting professor at the Society for the Humanities at Cornell University in Ithaca, New York, and author of *Deep Play*.

"Play always has a sacred place, some version of a playground, in which it happens. This place may be a classroom, a sports stadium, a stage, a courtroom, a coral reef, a workbench in a garage, a church or temple."

With so many playgrounds, it seems a crime against femininity to deny ourselves the chance to zip down the slide, so to speak. But if you need *reasons* to play, read on.

Play energizes. When you're intensely focused on play—building a Victorian dollhouse, cooking an elegant gourmet meal, digging in the garden—you're transported into a heightened and pleasant mental state called flow.

When you're in flow, you forget yourself. Time doesn't exist. You *become* your play: There is only this wood, this sauce, this dirt. You emerge from your trance refreshed and reenergized.

Play calms. While exercise and meditation are time-honored stress busters, a brief bout of play—mental or physical—can be just as effective.

Studies on the play habits of lab rats suggest that play may help rodents withstand environmental stressors—and that it may serve the same function in people, Dr. Ackerman notes.

"The parts of the brain that are thought to regulate play in rats are very similar to what we see in the human brain," says Steven Siviy, Ph.D., associate professor of psychology at Gettysburg College in Pennsylvania. "Rats who play as juveniles tend to deal better with social stressors—say, confronting another rat—as adults. So it's possible that play makes rats—and people—more adaptable and flexible," qualities that function as built-in stress buffers.

Play feels good. "When people play, there is a sense of good-humored, spirited, even sparkling pleasure," says Dr. Terr.

One woman, a writer and personal trainer in her late twenties, says she loves to play so much she's structured her life around it. "I compete in and write about sports as an excuse to play."

Some of us return to our childhood "playgrounds" later in life. Take Annette Bunge, Ph.D., a professor of chemical engineering in Golden, Colorado.

"I had to get over the idea that every minute of my life had to be productive," she says. Now she knows that her "play breaks" make her happier, more well-rounded, and more vital. So she's rediscovered the pleasures of running through sprinklers, riding the shopping carts at the grocery store, and sliding down stair banisters.

The Four Golden Rules of Play

If you haven't played in a while, you may not know where to start. Do you buy a hula hoop? Ride a roller-coaster?

Relax. It doesn't matter what you do, as long as you approach play with the right mindset. These guidelines will help define the rules of the game, whatever your game happens to be.

Make play dates—and keep them. "You must consciously *decide* to play," says Dr. Terr. So, as silly as it may seem, schedule regular play periods into your appointment book.

"My vision is for all adults to dedicate at least 1 percent of their life to play," says David Earl Platts, Ph.D., founder of David E. Platts and Associates, a management training, personal coaching, and counseling firm in England. "In practical terms, that's 15 minutes a day or less than 2 hours once a week."

Look to your past. Can't think of a thing that seems like fun? Think back to how—and what—you played as a girl. "You'll find clues as to what would be fun for you now," says Dr. Terr.

Say you loved playing with dolls. "You might collect dolls, make dollhouses, or fix old dolls," she says. You were the tomboy type? Consider signing up for the local women's softball or basketball league.

One 35-year-old woman remembered how she loved to play "pioneer" as a girl, creating her Wild West world with Lincoln Logs, dolls, and a little cast-iron cookstove. "Now that I'm grown, I've created my own little homestead on 1 acre, with chickens, bunnies, a greenhouse, gardens, and a woodstove," she says. "I guess some people never grow up."

A 36-year-old remembers the joy of coloring as a child. Once in college, when she began to experience stress, she remembered a friend's mother having told her that coloring helped with stress. Today, she says, "I still color. I find that I'm able to completely forget everything else. And when I'm done, I feel better."

Stay in the moment. To truly play, you must be able to put reality on hiatus. This means no composing a mental shopping list while you build that cute birdhouse you found in a crafts magazine. "If we don't live in the moment, how can we play with the moment?" says Sister Anne Bryan Smollin, C.S.J., Ph.D., executive director of Counseling for Laity in Albany, New York, and author of *Tickle Your Soul: Live Well, Love Much, Laugh Often.*

Says one 31-year-old woman: "I know I'm playing when I don't care about anything other than being in that exact moment. Like when I play with my dog. I stare at her, rub her belly, run around the backyard with her. When I'm doing that, I can't imagine anything else being that fun. But then we turn on the sprinkler. Oh, boy!"

Nix the I'm-not-good-enoughs. Some of us worry that we won't play "well." Perhaps we'd like to paint but can't draw a straight line, or we want to play volleyball but are embarrassed to try.

Fear of ridicule or failure kills playfulness dead, says Bernie DeKoven, a former toy designer and author of *The Well-Played Game*, who gives presentations on how to make work and play more fun.

Say you've never painted before and you want to give it a try. Great! But say you also think that the fruit bowl on your canvas must look exactly like the fruit bowl on your table. That's not fun. That's frustration.

Painting becomes play when you tune in to the "dance" between what you intend the painting to be and what it winds up being, says DeKoven. "That's the fun of it!"

Ready, Set, Play!

Dr. Terr once had a patient who found a stuffed animal in a cabin that she rents. "Weasel" has been her constant companion ever since.

Because the woman is a frequent traveler, Weasel has been to a great many places. He's washable, serves as a pillow on planes, and sits on the bed of every hotel room she has booked. People talk to him, and he talks back.

Someday, this young executive says, she's going to write a children's book about him.

This is a woman who's given herself *permission* to play. And if she can talk to a stuffed animal, you can approach play as a vast frontier filled with opportunities to revitalize your life.

Looking for new ways to play? Consider the ideas below for inspiration. But try anything and everything, from crossword puzzles and word games to kayaking and swing dancing. Trying on different types of play can help you define who you are, as well as what you might like to be.

Just as it did when you were a kid.

Turn Your Job into a Playground

Who says work has to be dull? Here's how to liven it up.

- Buy a Nerf gun (they're about 10 bucks at Kmart), and encourage your coworkers to do the same. Institute a new work ritual: Welcome new employees with an all-in-fun "ambush."
- Buy a small basketball hoop and a Nerf basketball. Place them in a quiet corner, away from others' workspace. When you hit your midafternoon energy slump, round up a few coworkers for a 15-minute game of Nerf basketball.
- Buy an Etch-a-Sketch and give yourself a daily artistic challenge. You might try to do a semirecognizable self-portrait in 5 minutes, "sketch" an item on your desk, or simply squiggle to your heart's content.
- Post one silly to-do on your appointment calendar or scheduling software. At 11:15 A.M. on Wednesday, write "Save world from meteor." At 2:58 P.M. on Thursday, "Disassemble computer; replace gerbil; reassemble computer." You get the idea.
- Buy a yo-yo that comes with an instruction booklet. When you're bored or stressed out, practice "walking the dog" for 10 minutes.

Make a Play Date with Your Mate

Put a little spark back in your marriage.

- Rent a convertible for a day and go for a long drive on a country road. Take a blanket and an armful of your favorite CDs. Stop at roadside antique stores. Rent a canoe for an hour. Continue on your merry way.
- Challenge your man to a game of strip poker. (If you're pathetic at cards, wear layers to prolong the

Create a Home Spa

When you can't escape to an exclusive spa by the sea, luxuriate at home. Here's how, says Laura Hittleman, beauty director of Canyon Ranch spa in Massachusetts.

Set the Stage

- Send your husband on a two-day trip with his pals. Let your kids stay with their friends or your parents. This weekend is all about you.
- Unplug the television and phone. Open your windows so you can hear nature—or play a nature sounds CD or soothing music.
- Post a picture of a place you've always wanted to visit where you can see it from your bathtub.
- Surround yourself with objects that give you strength, such as photos of your family.
- Turn off all overhead lights. Dim lamps or use colored lightbulbs. Light lots of candles.
- Buy a bouquet of your favorite flowers. (Ask the florist for extra petals—use them in your tub.)
- Get rid of clutter. Hide piles of bills and anything else that could stress you out.

Pamper Yourself

Try each of the following at least once over the weekend.

Have a hot-oil treatment. Warm ¼ cup of olive oil and 3 to 5 drops of essential oil (such as geranium, tea

fun.) Or drag out that dusty game of Twister—loser buys dinner.

- Shop together and ask him to give you a ride on the shopping cart. The disapproving stares of other grown-ups as you careen through aisle 7 are priceless.

tree, or peppermint). Massage into your scalp and cover with a plastic cap. Leave in hair for 30 minutes; then shampoo.

Bathe like a queen. Pour ½ cup of milk into your bathwater. Wrap a sliced orange in cheesecloth and squeeze under water to release the orange oil. Strew flower petals in the water, or add 5 or 6 drops of a relaxing essential oil (such as lavender) or vanilla extract.

Enjoy a facial. Chill ¼ cup aloe gel. Stir in the contents of a vitamin E capsule and ½ teaspoon vanilla extract; whip until frothy. Spread on your face for 10 to 15 minutes. Rinse with warm water. Place warm, moist chamomile tea bags on your eyes while you relax with the facial.

Don't stop there. Dry off with a big, fluffy cotton towel. Pull back your hair and slip on loose cotton clothing and comfortable shoes or thick socks. Then treat yourself to a manicure and pedicure. If you don't have cuticle cream, use olive oil.

Dine In

- Do all your shopping and prep work ahead of time.
- Dine on fresh fruit and vegetables, fish or chicken, whole-grain bread, and a light starch like couscous or rice. Have sorbet with sliced fruit for dessert.
- Keep a large bottle of springwater at your fingertips.

- Play the name game on car trips. You name a famous person. Your partner then has to come up with a celebrity whose name begins with the last letter of the name you gave. "My husband and I can play this for, oh, up to 7 hours—we're easily amused," says one woman.

Reenergizing Ways to Play with Friends

Let your pals in on the fun.

- Organize book-group dinner parties with meals from the month's novel. For example, if you're reading *Bridget Jones's Diary*, make shepherd's pie and smoothies (served with chardonnay, of course).
- Start "e-mail jousts" at work. One-upping each other's witticisms is a great way to get your creative juices flowing and to stay connected. Or challenge your friends to compose a haiku on a particular topic—say, spam.
- Cajole your mom, sister, neighbor, and a few good friends and coworkers to meet at the bowling alley every Wednesday night. Have everyone buy a bowling shirt, and arrange to have your names stitched on them.
- If there's a wildlife sanctuary near your home, take an all-day hike with a friend. Pack a fabulous lunch and take binoculars.
- If you sew, propose to some fellow needleworkers that you stage a weekly quilting bee or sewing circle.

10 Ways to Play Solo in 10 Minutes or Less

Nobody else around? No problem.

- While you wait in line at Wal-Mart, ponder playful questions. Examples: If people could fly . . . If men could give birth . . . What would the guy in front of me do if his wife sent him out to buy tampons?
- Pick up two oranges from the bowl on the kitchen table. Try to juggle. Juggle badly. Try three. Juggle even worse. Giggle. Start over. Repeat.
- Go fly a kite. Literally.

- Borrow your kids' blocks and try to build your dream house.
- Learn by heart a poem you've always loved.
- If it's summer, do some quick-and-dirty gardening before you take your morning shower.
- If there's snow on the ground, make a snow angel. Don't get up immediately. Look up at the clouds and see what they remind you of.
- Walk in the rain. Wear a pair of ratty sneakers so you can jump in a mud puddle if you feel like it.

Get Away from It All

A vacation should be all play and no work. But if yours turn into sightseeing marathons that leave you exhausted, try a new approach. In true Letterman style, here are the top 10 ways to have a relaxing vacation.

10. Let the kids help plan. There'll be less moping and complaining at tour sites if they agree with the vacation agenda. Stay at hotels with a swimming pool for the kids and a spa for you. Try to find activities for them that don't require your presence, so you can have some time to yourself or with your husband. Or, you and your husband can alternate who gets to sun by the pool and who gets to cart the kids around.

9. Leave the laptop and cell phone at home. Give your itinerary to one person at work in case of emergency, with strict instructions *not* to give it out. Resist the urge to check your voice mail. In fact, don't even buy the newspaper. You want to feel like you're living in a special world for at least these few days.

8. Spend within your means. While Hawaii is beautiful, it's a lot more fun if you can actually afford to buy food while you're there. Make sure you pick a destina-

tion or tour package that you can afford so you're not concerned about out-of-pocket expenses like meals and souvenirs.

7. Reserve the basics. Don't wait until you reach your destination to find a hotel or rent a car—especially if you're traveling with four or more people. You may end up with a single room or a compact car. Book everything in advance to reduce any possibility of anxiety-provoking uncertainty. While you're at it, buy your museum and transport passes, too.

6. Pin your kids. Nothing's more stressful than losing a kid in a strange town or country. Before leaving your room each day, pin your hotel's business card to the inside of your child's clothing—preferably to a layer they won't strip off and possibly lose when warm.

5. Learn the local currency and some key phrases. Find out the approximate equivalent of $10 in the local currency so you can make quick conversions while shopping. The exchange rate may change while you're away, but at least you'll have a general guide. Consider carrying a key-phrases book, too. This can help with ordering food, finding help, and so forth.

4. Watch for warnings. When traveling abroad, work with a travel agent to avoid problems related to local customs and to receive forewarning of major holidays that make it difficult to get basic services. Before you leave for vacation, ask your travel agent about any travel warnings related to your destination, and be mindful of potential health hazards related to foodborne or waterborne diseases. (In most foreign countries, it's a good idea to avoid the water.)

3. Leave your itinerary behind. You'll have greater peace of mind if you give your itinerary to someone who is watching your house or checking your mail. This way

you'll know that if any problems arise, someone can reach you.

2. Be flexible. It's good to have a plan, but remember, it won't be the end of the world if you don't stick to it exactly.

And the number-one way to have a relaxing vacation?

1. Vacation after your vacation. Arriving home late Sunday night only to get up early for work the next morning can smother your newfound vacation Zen. Instead, plan on coming home on a Saturday so you have a day to enjoy feeling relaxed before heading back to the office.

Energy Enhancing: 1 Year Later

It's 9:30 P.M., and Carolyn is nestled in a warm bath, thinking. It's been a year of change and renewed energy. She's filled her office with plants and the rejuvenating aroma of citrus. She's eating breakfast every morning and taking a walk every evening. She's started on a small dose of supplementary estrogen to help with some of her perimenopausal symptoms, joined a women's soccer team for fun, and chucked 15 years' worth of clutter from her house.

Of course, life occasionally knocks her off course, and her newfound vitality flags. That's when she must struggle to honor her energy enhancer bill of rights, which is still posted on her refrigerator at home and on her computer at work. But those times are fewer and further between.

She's learned to live by what she's come to call Carolyn's Credo: I Can't Do It All, and I Won't. She knows that a little self-care today is worth a ton of energy tomorrow.

Most of all, Carolyn has brought balance to her life, learned to live less hectically, learned to enjoy the moments when everything is going right and to work through the moments when things go wrong.

Yes, Carolyn's life is still stressful, but the days when she felt completely frustrated and helpless are gone. She now has control over her life and the energy to enjoy every day.

Index

Underscored page references indicate boxed text.